The ULTIMATE GUIDE TO INTERMITTENT FASTING

Burn Fat Quickly
with the Mini-Fast Diet

JULIAN WHITAKER, MD
and Peggy Dace

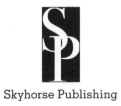

Skyhorse Publishing

Contents

Part III: Exercise and Diet Strategies

Acknowledgments

First and foremost, we would like to acknowledge Mark McCarty, the researcher who originally came up with the concept of the mini-fast with exercise. Mark's clinical trials (in conjunction with Babak Bahadori, MD), scientific papers, and enthusiasm inspired us to first test and then adopt this unique program at the Whitaker Wellness Institute.

The Whitaker Wellness physicians and staff, whose care and guidance have not only helped hundreds of our patients reap the benefits of this program, have also assisted in shaping and refining the Mini-Fast Diet. Special thanks to those who made the clinic's mini-fast study possible, particularly Shahana Faridi, who had the formidable task of organizing and tracking all study participants, Susie Heald, and Mark McCarty.

Healthy Directions, the company that has published *Health & Healing* every month for the last 21 years, has also been instrumental in getting this message out to hundreds of thousands of readers and for organizing the Diabesity Challenge, which provided further proof of the program's efficacy. To Ashley Delaney, Jennifer Myers, Jamie Whaley, Donna Engelgau, Michael Liebergot, and the entire Healthy Directions team, thanks.

As for the book itself, we are grateful for Ryann Smith Groseclose's editing and other contributions, and for the talented and gracious women at Rodale Books: Anne Egan, who was key in getting this project off the ground and editors Bridget Doherty, Karen Bolesta, Andrea Au Levitt, and Nancy Fitzgerald. And as always, a special note of gratitude goes to our families for their love, patience, and understanding.

Finally—and perhaps most important—we thank all of the participants in the mini-fast study at Whitaker Wellness, the *Health & Healing* Diabesity Challenge, and everyone else who has used this program to achieve their health goals. We are especially appreciative of those who generously shared their personal stories: Mary Olson, Elizabeth Billups, Don Engmann, Roxie Tanner, Stephanie and Jack Pacheco, John Sorci, Galen Clayton, Bill Barbic, Brian Shook, Michael Carney, Susie Heald, Barbara Hauth, Sue Anderson, Robert Geiger, Bob Ewing, Sarah Dela Cruz, Connie Whitaker, Harry Willwater, Cindy Lumpkin, and all the others who preferred to go by first name or initials only. Your successes, which inspire and motivate others, are the heart and soul of this book.

Introduction

When I was growing up in the 1950s—the prehistoric days before video games and a TV in every room— kids spent most of their spare time running around outdoors. We played pickup games of baseball, shot hoops in the driveway, tossed footballs in the front yard, and hung out all day at the swimming pool in the summer. When we couldn't go outside, my brothers and I would bring our games inside and drive our mom crazy with all our roughhousing. Back then, fat kids were few and far between.

In junior high and high school, I participated in basketball, football, and track, and played football in college. I've run seven marathons and more 10-Ks than I can remember. For a few years I was into cycling, and in 1995, I rode a bike across the country, 4,300 miles in 10 weeks. Tennis, racquetball, squash: I've played them all. My wife, Connie, who is a dyed-in-the-wool exerciser, and I have also always had various pieces of exercise equipment, most of them that she purchased. Although I've never been a skinny guy—I'm definitely a mesomorph, big boned and fairly muscular—I never had a weight problem, either.

About 15 years ago, I slowed down. I didn't just sit on the couch. I golfed, did a little walking and jogging, and occasionally hiked and played sports with my kids. But somehow I lost the urge to work out for exercise's sake. And I gained weight. Of course, my diet had something to do with it. I've always had a big appetite, but with my former degree of activity, it didn't seem to matter. Once I became less active, however, I guess I forgot to tell my appetite, and the weight just kept piling on.

I didn't like it one bit. I tried cutting calories, slashing my fat intake, reducing carbohydrates, and going on exercise binges. I would lose 5 to 10 pounds, but I'd always gain them back—and a couple of extras to boot. I finally topped out at about 250 pounds, which, mesomorph or not, was way too much for my 6-foot frame. It was embarrassing! I looked like the Michelin Man.

Then I learned about the mini-fast with exercise, the program that is the cornerstone of this book. From a scientific and medical perspective, it made perfect sense, so I decided to try it. Although I understood from a biochemical perspective why this program burns fat and reduces appetite, I was nevertheless surprised at how well it worked. I used to be ravenous after exercising. On the mini-fast I wasn't even hungry, and I had no trouble waiting until noon to eat. I also liked the fact that, because I was cutting out a meal, I didn't have to worry about counting calories or "dieting."

I began losing weight the very first week. Success, as the saying goes, breeds success, and this motivated me to stay on the program. Before I knew it, I had lost 10 pounds, then 15, then 20. I told the six other doctors at the Whitaker Wellness Institute, my clinic in Newport Beach, California, about the mini-fast with exercise, and they began prescribing it to their patients, many of whom also saw results right away. I wrote about it in my monthly newsletter, *Health & Healing*, and it generated so much interest that we ran a "Biggest Loser" contest, which provided additional feedback on the program's ease and efficacy. (You'll read many of their success stories in this book.)

I'm telling you my personal experience—and, believe me, I'm not crazy about advertising my struggles with weight—because I hope that it will motivate you to look at this book as not just another diet gimmick. The mini-fast with exercise is the most effective weight loss program I've seen in my nearly 40 years of practicing medicine. My purpose in writing *The Ultimate Guide to Intermittent Fasting* is to get this valuable information into the hands of those who need and want to lose weight but just can't make it happen.

Many of you reading this would like to drop a few pounds so you'll look and feel better, and that's a laudable goal. But you also need to realize the toll that excess weight takes on your health. Obesity, which affects one in three Americans, is the most significant medical challenge our country is facing today. Weight loss not only makes you look terrific and feel good about yourself, but it's also a powerful therapy for preventing, treating, and reversing a broad range of serious health problems.

Even if you've been unsuccessful in your past attempts to get a handle on your weight, I urge you to give the Mini-Fast Diet a try. As I said, it is, hands down, the most successful, health-enhancing, and fastest-acting weight loss program I've ever come across. It eliminates the restrictive diets, calorie counting, and food cravings that are the bane of most regimens. It promotes habits that will lead to a lifetime of health. And it delivers the single most important result that all dieters want but few other approaches specifically target—it selectively burns fat.

Wishing you the best on your quest for optimal health,
Julian Whitaker, MD

PART I

The Problem— And the Solution

I have had metabolic syndrome for at least 20 years. When I started on your program, my weight was 265. Now, less than 3 months later, it's 248—a drop of 17 pounds—and I am keeping it off without a struggle, just with a commitment to follow this simple regimen. My appetite is reduced; I rarely even want anything before lunch; and I eat less for lunch and dinner as well. I have no doubt I will reach my weight loss goal within several months. Thank you for showing me the way to manage my metabolic syndrome.

—H.N., ATLANTA

CHAPTER 1

WHY MOST DIETS FAIL

The second day of a diet is always easier than the first. By the second day, you're off it.

—JACKIE GLEASON

If you're trying to lose weight, the last thing you need is another book that tells you to eat less and exercise more—you already know that. Except for the very small minority of people whose metabolism lets them eat whatever they want and never gain a pound, you're going to have to burn more calories than you take in if you want to lose weight. Furthermore, once you hit that magic number, you'll have to keep your activity level up and your calorie intake down, or you'll be back at square one before you know it.

Yet these are the two stumbling blocks in virtually every weight loss endeavor, whether it's a plan you've read in a book or online, a commercial program, or you're simply going it on your own. You get hungry or you feel the diet is overly restrictive, so you cheat or give it up altogether. Regular exercise is too time-consuming or too boring, and you stop working out. Once again, you're disappointed with the promises of easy weight loss that didn't pan out. Above all, you're disappointed with your own failings.

Don't be too hard on yourself. Being overweight doesn't mean you're self-indulgent, lazy, or undisciplined. Obesity isn't a character flaw. If you eat too much and find it a chore to lace up your walking shoes, you're just following your natural instincts.

IT'S NOT YOUR FAULT

For millions of years, our ancestors were hunters and gatherers. Because they endured cycles of feast and famine, survival depended on seeking out the most high-calorie, energy-dense foods available—and when they were fortunate enough to find them, eating like there was no tomorrow. Thus, we are genetically programmed to be attracted to and indiscriminately eat calorie-rich fare.

Animals' eating habits are also dictated by their DNA, so why aren't they fat? Imagine the spectacle of squirrels in your local park with puffy cheeks and potbellies so big they can't even climb trees. Squirrels and other animals in the wild aren't thin and lively because they're disciplined. It's because the effort required for them to obtain food has remained more or less constant throughout history. With domesticated animals, it's a different story. Siamese cats and cocker spaniels did not evolve on a diet of table scraps and canned meat, and survival required more than moseying over to the food dish a couple of times a day. But that's the situation most household pets find themselves in today, and as a result, half of the dogs and cats in this country are obese.

It's the same with humans. Until the relatively recent past, food was scarce, and high-calorie foods were few and far between. A great deal of physical effort was required to get enough calories to stay alive, let alone to gain excess weight. The modern world is a radical departure from that environment. We no longer have to hunt or gather, unless you consider shopping for groceries "gathering." In fact, food practically stalks us! It beckons us from our fridges and cupboards, the break room at work, drive-thrus and shopping centers, in magazines and on TV. Everywhere we turn we're enticed by the sights and smells of food.

And much of it is high-calorie fare—precisely what we are hardwired to want. If you had to choose between a bountiful salad and a bowl of rocky road ice cream with whipped cream on top, which would you find more attractive? If you are honest and go for the ice cream as most would, you're simply following your genetic impulses to maximize your caloric intake. Some experts like to pin the obesity crisis on food manufacturers for providing fatty, sugary, processed foods or on restaurants for serving supersize portions. But these businesses would go broke if all they offered was spinach and tomatoes. They're just giving us what we want.

I could make a similar case for exercise, or rather the near universal aversion to exercise. I'm not saying our DNA promotes laziness, but there is an inborn drive to conserve energy. It's human nature to do what needs to be done and not much more. The tendency for most people—whether it's work, chores around the house, or physical activities—is to do just enough to get by. If a task that requires exertion isn't motivated by reward or punishment (exercise is a prime example), it's less likely to get done.

If you want to see our natural, calorie-maximization, energy-conservation instincts in action, go to an all-you-can-eat buffet, or sit down to a holiday dinner. Watch cars circle around a store's parking lot as drivers jockey for spots near the entrance, or count the number of people who take the stairs versus an escalator. To gauge the impact of these behaviors, visit the mall, a sporting or cultural event, or another public gathering, and take

WHAT WE EAT

Between 1971 and 2000, our average daily caloric intake increased by 335 calories for women (1,542 to 1,877) and by 168 for men (2,450 to 2,618).[1] Since then, calorie counts have remained relatively stable and may have even decreased a bit. There's also been a slight decline in the percentage of total calories from carbohydrates, although it still hovers at around 50 percent, with 16 percent from protein and 34 percent from fat.[2] The most significant dietary change over the past 4 decades is that we are getting more and more of our calories from added sugars, fats, soft drinks, and "mixtures of mainly grain" in "prepared, frozen, and take-out meal combinations"[3]—high-calorie foods that pack on the pounds, wreak havoc on blood sugar levels, and make losing weight all the more difficult.

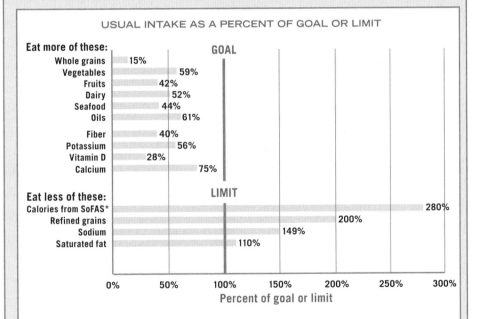

USUAL INTAKE AS A PERCENT OF GOAL OR LIMIT

Eat more of these:

Whole grains	15%
Vegetables	59%
Fruits	42%
Dairy	52%
Seafood	44%
Oils	61%
Fiber	40%
Potassium	56%
Vitamin D	28%
Calcium	75%

Eat less of these:

Calories from SoFAS*	280%
Refined grains	200%
Sodium	149%
Saturated fat	110%

Percent of goal or limit

* SoFAS = solid fats and added sugars

Note: Bars show average intakes for all individuals (ages 1 or 2 years or older, depending on the data source) as a percent of the recommended intake level or limit. Recommended intakes for food groups and limits for refined grains and solid fats and added sugars are based on amounts in the USDA 2,000-calorie food pattern. Recommended intakes for fiber, potassium, vitamin D, and calcium are based on the highest AI or RDA for ages 14 to 70 years. Limits for sodium are based on the UL and for saturated fat on 10% of calories. The protein foods group is not shown here because, on average, intake is close to recommended levels.

Based on data from: U.S. Department of Agriculture, Agricultural Research Service and U.S. Department of Health and Human Services, Centers for Disease Control and Prevention. What We Eat in America, NHANES 2001–2004 or 2005–2006.

a look at the crowd. Two-thirds of the people walking around have a weight problem.

Bottom line: Don't beat yourself up if you're overweight. It's not your fault. Just recognize that because losing weight requires you to work against your natural instincts, it's going to take a little more effort and discipline on your part—which is why you need a scientifically proven, patient-tested, no-gimmicks guide like the Mini-Fast Diet.

THE DIET INDUSTRY: WHAT WORKS?

At any given time, 75 million Americans are dieting, and there is no shortage of offers to help. According to the latest edition of *The U.S. Weight Loss & Diet Control Market,* published by Market-data Enterprises, we are expected to spend $66.5 billion per year in our quest to get thin.[4]

The weight loss market includes commercial programs such as Weight Watchers, Jenny Craig, and TOPS (Take Off Pounds Sensibly), and medically supervised clinics that specialize in weight reduction. It encompasses prepared foods from companies such as Nutrisystem, as well as meal replacement shakes and bars from Slim-Fast and dozens of other manufacturers. There are books that tell you how to drop pounds by eating low-carb with plenty of meat, or by going high-carb vegetarian or vegan. You can diet according to your blood type, your metabolic type, and even your zodiac sign, or you can eat like a caveman, a Frenchwoman, or a movie star. Cabbage soup, grapefruit, apple cider vinegar, lemonade, beer, cookies, chocolate—the range of weight loss angles out there is truly remarkable.

What if I were to tell you that you could lose weight on most any diet? It's true, provided that you actually follow the diet.

Regardless of the hook or gimmick, virtually every plan has one thing in common: They all require you to eat fewer calories (yes, even the chocolate and cookie diets). I'm not saying that they're all equally nutritious or advisable, only that the crux of weight loss, for most people, is calorie restriction.

Proponents of various programs will say that their way is the only way, and they may even be able to produce evidence to back up their claims. But, remember, just because someone's brother lost 30 pounds on one diet, or a celebrity slimmed down on another, isn't proof positive—few of these approaches have ever been subjected to scientific scrutiny. Yet the studies that have been conducted demonstrate that a variety of diets do indeed work, at least over the short term.

One representative study is a British clinical trial that compared four well-known programs: the Atkins low-carb diet, Slim-Fast's regimen of low-calorie meal replacements, Weight Watchers' point system for calorie control plus weekly meetings, and Rosemary Conley's regimen of a low-fat diet and weekly group exercise classes, which is popular in the United Kingdom. Researchers enrolled 300 overweight or obese participants, assigned equal numbers to each program, and followed them for 6 months.

All of the participants lost a similar amount of weight and body fat regardless of the diet they were on. The average loss was 13 pounds total and 9 pounds of fat. The group following the Atkins diet lost more during the first 4 weeks, but the other approaches were equally effective over the 6-month study period.

The Rest of the Story

Here's the rest of the story. These people had every chance of success. As with all clinical trials, the selection process was arduous. The volunteers had an excellent support system and were communicated with regularly, as often as once a week for those in programs that included meetings or classes. They were reimbursed for classes, books, meal replacements, travel expenses, and other related costs, and they were offered a free diet of their choice at the study's conclusion. Yet 28 percent dropped out of the study. They claimed that the diet was intolerable. They weren't losing enough weight. Or they simply stopped showing up. Whatever the excuse, more than a quarter of these highly motivated, well-supported people couldn't stay on a diet for 6 months.

Even more telling, participants were asked to be reevaluated 6 months later. Only 54 percent complied with this request, and at that point their dieting behavior had changed dramatically. Fewer than half were still on their original diets; the others had swapped programs or were dieting on their own. (More people stuck with or switched to the group-based approaches.) At the end, 20 people remained in Weight Watchers, 20 in Rosemary Conley, 9 in Atkins, and 9 in Slim-Fast. Although these small numbers limit statistical analysis, the researchers concluded that individuals who stayed with a diet for 1 year sustained an average weight loss of 10 percent of their initial body mass.[5]

Similar results were seen in a 2-year study published in 2010. Researchers from Temple University in Philadelphia pitted a low-fat diet against a low-carbohydrate one, both in combination with an intensive lifestyle modification program that included regular exercise and group support. The average weight loss on both diets was nearly identical, about 11 percent of baseline at 6 and at 12 months. After 2 years, however, some of the weight had crept back on, and at the study's conclusion, the mean loss was 7 percent. In this study there also was a fair amount of falloff. After a year, about a quarter of participants failed to return for assessment, and at the 2-year mark, 32 percent of the low-fat group and 42 percent of the low-carb group had dropped out.[6]

Let's push that date out 4 or 5 years. How successful are dieters at that point? The data is pretty grim. When a research team at UCLA reviewed 31 studies of long-term outcomes of various calorie-restricting programs in order to determine which were the most effective, they found that up to two-thirds of the dieters had regained more weight than they lost while dieting.[7] You don't need a scientific study to tell you this. You've probably seen it

WHAT ABOUT DRUGS?

Weight loss is the holy grail of the pharmaceutical industry. Who wouldn't love to stay skinny simply by popping a pill? Just imagine the sales! So far, Big Pharma has failed to come up with a medication that's both effective and safe.

You may remember fen-phen, a drug combo (fenfluramine and phentermine) that was taken off the market in 1997 after it was linked with increased risk of heart valve problems and pulmonary hypertension. Because the cardiovascular issues were actually associated with fenfluramine, phentermine is still available as an appetite suppressant. It can take the edge off hunger, but its efficacy levels off over time, there's a potential for addiction, and it has numerous adverse effects, including increased blood pressure and heart rate. Fat blockers are another class of weight loss meds. Orlistat (Xenical and Alli) inhibits enzymes that digest fat, causing about 30 percent of the fat you eat to pass through the intestinal tract rather than being absorbed. Not surprisingly, these medications are notorious for unpleasant side effects such as diarrhea, gas, oily spotting on underwear, and difficulty controlling bowel movements, as well as impaired absorption of fat-soluble vitamins.

In 2012, the FDA approved two new weight loss drugs: Qsymia (a combination of phentermine and topiramate, an anticonvulsant medication) and Belviq (lorcaserin, an appetite suppressant). These drugs have numerous side effects—and both were rejected earlier due to safety concerns. Don't hold your breath waiting for a pill that enables you to eat whatever you want and never gain weight. The benefits of all diet drugs are modest, and this approach does nothing to improve long-term weight management.

among your circle of friends, and certainly with the celebrities whose weight fluctuations are mercilessly chronicled in the media. No doubt about it, long-term weight maintenance is tough.

I'm not telling you this to discourage you or to disparage other programs; rather, I'm simply trying to inject a dose of reality into the diet debate. There's a saying, "The best diet is the one you stick to." But as these studies—and, most likely, your personal experience—illustrate, that's the problem. It may not matter which program you select or what combination of fat, protein, and carbohydrate you eat, but your compliance with your chosen program is of the utmost importance.

SECRETS OF SUCCESSFUL LOSERS

We've established that most people who try to lose weight are unsuccessful. Either they're unable to take off pounds in the first place or they gain them back over time. But some individuals break that mold. I have patients who've been coming to Whitaker Wellness for annual checkups who've maintained their fighting weight for 15, 20, and even 25 years. What makes them and others like them different?

To answer this question, researchers from the University of Colorado and Brown Medical School have been studying the strategies, behaviors, and other characteristics of people who have lost weight and kept it off. In 1994, they established the National Weight Control Registry (NWCR), which has tracked more than 5,000 men and women who have achieved and maintained their optimal weight. Weight losses range from 30 to 300 pounds, and maintenance periods span from 1 to nearly 70 years, with averages of 66 pounds and 5½ years.

The NWCR isn't a weight loss program, nor does it espouse a particular approach. Some of these people lost weight rapidly, while others took years to do it. Fifty-five percent followed a program of some sort, and the remainder made up their own rules. Regardless of this diversity, however, successful losers have a few things in common:

- 98 percent modified their food intake
- 94 percent increased their physical activity
- To keep the weight off, most of these people continue to eat a low-calorie, low-fat diet

Other behaviors frequently associated with optimal weight maintenance include:

- 90 percent exercise, an average of an hour a day; walking is the most popular activity
- 75 percent weigh themselves at least once a week
- 62 percent watch fewer than 10 hours of television a week[8]

WHAT MAKES THE MINI-FAST DIET DIFFERENT

The only way to achieve enduring weight loss is to eat right and exercise more, and that's exactly what the Mini-Fast Diet is all about. It's a program that makes cutting calories easier and exercise, well, if not painless, then definitely more rewarding. The mini-fast with exercise, as we call it, is a proven protocol that has been studied in clinical trials. It has been adopted by thousands of people, some of whom you'll read about in this book. And it's the primary weight loss program at my clinic, the Whitaker Wellness Institute in Newport Beach, California.

When I opened the clinic in 1979, many of my patients struggled with their weight, but obesity was rare and extreme obesity virtually unheard of. Since then, more than 50,000 patients have come to the clinic, and over that time I've observed firsthand obesity's insidious creep into our society and its adverse effects on our health. Although the treatment programs at Whitaker Wellness have always focused on nutrition, exercise, and other natural therapies—and many patients do well on this approach—obesity has become such an overwhelming problem that I realized I needed to come up with a more effective prescription for permanent weight loss.

I needed to figure out a strategy for reducing calories that would be less arduous. I was looking for an approach that would heighten the effects of exercise and selectively burn fat. I insisted that it be a lifestyle program that my patients could adopt and stick with, rather than a short-lived diet. And it had to be a regimen that could produce predictable results that were both rapid and lasting. When I came across the mini-fast with exercise, I intuitively knew that it was the answer. Today, after following hundreds of people who have enthusiastically embraced this plan—and losing 20 pounds myself—I can tell you without reservation that this is the most successful program for enduring weight loss ever.

We'll get into the details in subsequent chapters, but here's a synopsis of why this unique approach works.

Makes It Easier to Eat Less

Restricting calories, as we've discussed, is tough because it goes against human nature. Unfortunately, we've also established that in order to lose weight, you need to do just that. This program takes a big chunk out of your daily caloric intake because it eliminates one meal outright—that's the mini-fast portion. Believe it or not, this is much, much easier than counting calories and eating less throughout the day. We're all familiar with the "see-food diet," which some anonymous wit came up with: "You see food and you want to eat it." By skipping one meal per day, you're significantly lowering your overall calorie consumption without having to resist the temptation of overeating and making poor food choices, which we face at each and every meal.

I know this goes against the conventional wisdom that it's important to eat three meals a day and to never, ever miss breakfast, but as it turns out, that common admonition has no factual basis. As you'll see, this approach is scientifically based, clinically proven—and it works.

Takes the Edge Off Appetite

I know that many of you are thinking, "There's no way I can miss a meal. I'd just get too hungry." But the other aspects of the program—exercise and optional nutritional supplements—truly take the edge off appetite. You may have to try it and see for yourself, but when you skip breakfast, particularly if you've been eating the typical high-carb American breakfast of cereal, juice, pancakes, toast, etc., you'll say goodbye to the midmorning blood sugar lows that make you crave a snack and feel famished by lunchtime. And exercising while mini-fasting revs up physiological processes that further blunt appetite.

These comments from Lewis of Newport Beach echo the experience of most people who have adopted this program: "I can't believe how much this program reduces appetite. I drink coffee in the mornings, but I rarely think about food. In fact, sometimes I don't even think about lunch until somebody asks if I want to get something to eat. I've never felt like I was on a diet, but I've lost 16 pounds, down to where I need to be, and have no problem keeping them off."

Accommodates a Wide Range of Food Preferences

A common pitfall of many diets is that you grow tired of the allowed foods. The Atkins plan is a perfect example. I don't care how much you love meat, cheese, and eggs. Eating them day in and day out gets old. You crave variety, you miss your oranges and apples, or you feel you can't go another day without a piece of bread or a tortilla, so you cave in. The mini-fast with exercise accommodates all food preferences. Roxie, whom you'll read about in Chapter 4, is a vegan. Michael, in Chapter 11, is a meat-and-potatoes guy. Mary leans toward low-carb until dinner, and Mark eats a very low-fat diet. This program works equally well for all of them. Furthermore, no foods are strictly off-limits, so you don't have to deal with the "forbidden fruit syndrome" of wanting something all the more because you can't have it. If you're a chocoholic or a dessert lover, have some. Just be smart about it.

Please understand that I'm not suggesting you can skip one meal, then make up for those uneaten calories by eating with abandon the rest of the day. The people who get the most rapid and enduring results are those who eat a healthy, moderately low-fat, low-glycemic diet. Weight loss aside, this is a foundation of optimal health. However, as long as you don't go hog wild, anything goes. In Chapters 11 and 12, you'll find the nutritional guidelines we recommend at the Whitaker Wellness Institute, along with 67 delicious recipes. There's also a 2-week meal plan created by the professional nutritionists and chefs at the Rodale Test Kitchen. No matter what kinds of food you like, you'll find dishes that will entice your tastebuds.

Dramatically Enhances the Benefits of Exercise

Numerous studies have shown that exercise alone is not a particularly effective weight loss strategy. It takes a surprisingly large expenditure of energy to lose weight—an estimated 3,500 calories for every pound dropped. Nor does exercise burn as many calories as you may expect; for instance, walking for an hour at a robust 4 miles an hour burns 150 to 200 calories. Furthermore, research demonstrates that when people work out, there's usually a compensatory increase in caloric intake. All that activity makes us hungry, or we're consciously or subconsciously rewarding ourselves for exercising. Either way we tend to eat more.[9]

Let's say you're willing to go to the effort of working out—and make no mistake, it takes effort to begin and continue with an exercise program. You want to reap maximum benefits, right? That's where this program surpasses all others. If your goal is losing weight and burning fat, *when* you exercise is as important as *how much* you exercise. This is the real magic of the mini-fast with exercise regimen.

Selectively Burns Fat

Heavy people think they want to lose weight, but what they really want is to lose fat. If you exercise after eating, you'll use the carbohydrates from that meal for energy. But if you exercise during a mini-fasting period—especially in the morning after fasting overnight—when your carbohydrate stores are nearly depleted, your body has no choice but to start burning fat. Provided that you don't replace that fat you've lost by overeating the rest of the day, you'll be chipping away at your fat stores and seeing results in no time.

We're witnessing phenomenal reductions not only in weight but also in waist and hip circumference, as well as improvements in body composition on this program. Galen, for example, whose story is in Chapter 8, has been a committed exerciser for some time. Yet 12 weeks after starting on the mini-fast, exercising in the morning, and skipping breakfast, she lost 10 pounds of fat, 4 inches around her waist, and two dress sizes.

Includes a Fail-Safe Motivation System

Overcoming our natural inclination to eat too much and sit on the couch is the most difficult part of any weight loss attempt. The knowledge that you need to exercise and eat right, the desire to do so, and the perfect program to follow simply aren't enough. If they were, we wouldn't be experiencing the obesity problems we are today.

For 20 years I've been using what I call Instant Willpower to help my patients stick with their diets, exercise regularly, stop smoking, and change other unwanted behaviors. This system, which I'll explain in Chapter 6, helped Jose stop smoking and Raquel break her Diet Coke habit. It's helped me get up and exercise even on days when I would much rather have slept in, and is an integral contributor to my weight loss.

Has No Added Costs

You don't need to go out and buy a bunch of stuff to follow this program. Because exercise is a requirement, you will need a decent pair of shoes if you select walking as your activity, as most do, or whatever gear is needed, should you choose another activity. No special foods are required, and, in fact, you may save money on groceries, since you'll be eating one fewer meal per day. In Chapter 5, I'll tell you about two nutritional supplements that suppress appetite and facilitate fat burning, but they are strictly optional. Some of the people who have lost weight on this program take these supplements religiously, and others don't use them at all. If you do decide to try them, their purchase would, of course, be an additional expense.

Aside from the supplements, which I want to stress are by no means mandatory, there are no other costs—no meeting fees, no meal replacements, no gym memberships. All told, the mini-fast with exercise is not only the most valuable weight loss program I know of but also the least expensive.

Provides Broad Benefits Beyond Weight Loss

Weight loss is a reward in and of itself. However, this program gives you so much more. In addition to improving or eliminating type 2 diabetes, metabolic syndrome, and other obesity-related disorders, this unique approach turns on a number of genes and physiological mechanisms that reduce free radical activity, quell inflammation, increase resistance to disease—and even extend longevity.

Not a Diet but a Lifestyle

The only way to achieve lasting weight loss is to change your lifestyle, and change it for good. Once you start noticing results—and if you follow this program, you will see results—and realize how much easier it is than restrictive diets, I predict that you'll be encouraged to join the thousands of others who have made the mini-fast with exercise a permanent part of their lives. As Mary Olson, whose story you'll read on the next page, says: "What do you have to lose? Not money. Not time. Just the extra poundage!"

Mary Olson: "It's Made Me Feel Good in My Own Skin Again"

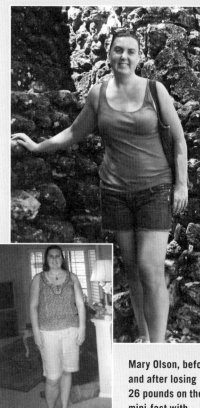

Mary Olson, before and after losing 26 pounds on the mini-fast with exercise program

Mary Olson practically grew up at the Whitaker Wellness Institute. During high school, she worked in our vitamin warehouse a couple of afternoons a week and transferred to the vitamin store when she was in college. After getting her degree in education, she left us for a few years to teach elementary school. Then the economic turndown led her back to us on a part-time basis—the school's loss but our gain. In 2010, we conducted a clinical trial of the mini-fast with exercise program at Whitaker Wellness (more on this study in Chapter 3) and invited our employees to participate. Mary was among the first to sign up. Here's her story.

"Over the past 8 years, I put on 30 pounds. I'm tall and carried it fairly well, but it really bothered me. I've tried many diets, including the Hollywood Miracle Diet, a modified Weight Watchers program, and even fen-phen. I'd lose 5 to 10 pounds, but I'd invariably gain the weight back. I was always searching for new ways to lose weight, and when Dr. Whitaker announced that he was looking for volunteers to participate in a study he was doing on the mini-fast, I thought, 'Why not give this a try?'

"So far I've lost 26 pounds, and gone from a size 14—with a muffin top—to a comfortable size 10! This program has really increased my exercise. I am a member of 24 Hour Fitness, although I used to rarely take advantage of my membership. Once I started on this program, however, I began working out there 3 days a week. I take group classes that include a cardio workout, a SET class (strength, endurance, and training—a mixture of cardio and weights), and Bodypump, which focuses solely on weight training. I also try to swim 1 or 2 days a week when possible. It's a little hard to always work out in the morning, since some of the classes I take are in the evenings after work. But I figure any time is better than never.

"I skip breakfast and only have my cup (or four) of coffee. Adjusting to no breakfast was hard the first couple of days—a grumbling stomach and headaches. But now it's second nature. For lunch I usually have a salad or protein of some sort, and try not to eat more than 5 grams of carbs. For dinner I have whatever I want. I don't like the deprivation that so many diets have, and I will never stick to a diet that makes me want for specific foods. I don't go crazy, but if I want a bowl of ice cream for dessert, I'll have it. Around 4:00 in the afternoon, I sometimes think about a snack, but I tell myself, 'Just wait until 6:00 and have all you want for dinner.' This is what works for me.

"As I said, I've lost 26 pounds. I'd like to lose 7 more pounds—then I won't be lying on my driver's license, which still states the weight I was at age 20. And I know I can do it. My health is great. I substitute-teach a couple of days a week, and I'm able to keep up with all the kiddos. And it's made me feel good in my own skin again. I love that I can go shopping and try on a size 10, and pretty soon *that* will be too big for me!

"I consider myself something of a diet expert, since I've tried so many. But this 'diet'—if you can call it that—is the first one I can actually see myself staying on for the rest of my life. I've already been on it for nearly a year, and for me it's so easy! It's a money saver, too, since I don't have to buy breakfast foods. I eat normally the other two meals of the day, so there are no 'special' foods to buy or meetings to attend. My advice for anyone considering the mini-fast with exercise would be to just try it. What do you have to lose? Not money. Not time. Just the extra poundage!"

CHAPTER 2

WHY WEIGHT LOSS MATTERS

If past obesity trends continue unchecked, the negative effects on the health of the U.S. population will increasingly outweigh the positive effects gained from declining smoking rates. Failure to address continued increases in obesity could result in an erosion of the pattern of steady gains in health observed since early in the 20th century.

—HARVARD INTERFACULTY PROGRAM
FOR HEALTH SYSTEMS IMPROVEMENT[1]

Whenever there is an abundance of easily accessible food, some people will get fat. It's inevitable. Historically, an expansive girth was considered a sign of prosperity, a display of one's ability to procure food even in times of scarcity. Think of Henry VIII, whose armor suggests that he had a 52-inch waist; the portly royalty of Hawaii; and "fat cats," a term coined in the 1920s to describe rich, influential men. In eras of economic stability and affordable food, there are a fair number of heavy people across all socioeconomic strata. The percentage of Americans who are overweight, about one in three, hasn't changed much since the government began tracking this trend more than 50 years ago.

The prevalence of obesity, however—defined as a body mass index (BMI) of 30 or higher or 20 percent above desirable weight (see Chapter 7 for more on BMI)—has more than doubled. From 1960 to the mid-1970s, it hovered around 14 to 15 percent, then began a steady climb, increasing by 24 percent between 2000 and

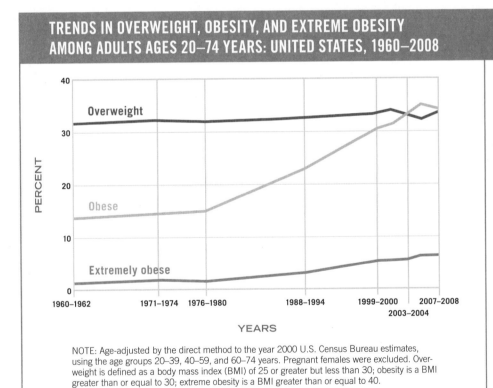

TRENDS IN OVERWEIGHT, OBESITY, AND EXTREME OBESITY AMONG ADULTS AGES 20–74 YEARS: UNITED STATES, 1960–2008

NOTE: Age-adjusted by the direct method to the year 2000 U.S. Census Bureau estimates, using the age groups 20–39, 40–59, and 60–74 years. Pregnant females were excluded. Overweight is defined as a body mass index (BMI) of 25 or greater but less than 30; obesity is a BMI greater than or equal to 30; extreme obesity is a BMI greater than or equal to 40.

SOURCE: CDC/NCHS, National Health Examination Survey cycle I (1960–1962); National Health and Nutrition Examination Survey I (1971–1974), II (1976–1980), and III (1988–1994), 1999–2000, 2001–2002, 2003–2004, 2005–2006, and 2007–2008.

2005 alone.[2] Severe, or morbid, obesity (a BMI of 40 or greater) barely registered until about 1980, when it, too, picked up speed. In the early to mid-2000s, the number of Americans with a BMI above 40 grew by 50 percent, and those with a BMI above 50 increased by 75 percent.[3] Today, obesity and overweight rates run neck and neck—or should I say belly and belly—at about 34 percent each, and severe obesity now affects approximately 6 percent of our population.

OBESITY'S WEIGHTY BURDEN

These trends have had and will continue to have dramatic effects on many facets of our society. Airlines struggle with seat sizes and extra fuel consumption incurred by widespread obesity, and the Federal Transit Administration, acknowledging the "expanding girth of the average passenger," recently proposed increasing the mean weight per bus passenger. Products ranging from 350-pound-capacity chairs and collapse-resistant toilets to oversize wheelchairs and jumbo caskets have come on the market. In addition to plus-size clothing stores, there are dating services and travel agencies that cater to heavy people and law firms that specialize in weight discrimination cases.

Obesity also has a major financial impact. In December 2010, the Society of Actuaries released a study that pegged the total costs of obesity in the United States and Canada at $300 billion a year (Americans account for 90 percent of this amount). This astronomical sum includes loss of productivity in the workplace due to disability ($43 billion), totally disabled workers ($72 billion), and premature death ($49 billion). The study also found that obesity and overweight added $127 billion in medical bills.[4] According to a report by John Cawley of Cornell University and Chad Meyerhoefer of Lehigh University, released in 2010 by the

WEIGHT-RELATED HEALTH CHALLENGES

✔ Metabolic syndrome

✔ Type 2 diabetes and its many complications

✔ Coronary heart disease

✔ Cancer of the colon, breast, endometrium, kidney, esophagus, and possibly other organs

✔ Hypertension

✔ Blood lipid abnormalities (high LDL cholesterol and triglycerides, low HDL cholesterol)

✔ Stroke

✔ Liver disease

✔ Kidney disease

✔ Gallbladder disease

✔ Sleep apnea

✔ Respiratory problems

✔ Osteoarthritis

✔ Gynecological problems (abnormal periods, infertility)

✔ Urinary incontinence

✔ Digestive disorders (gastroesophageal reflux disease, or heartburn)

✔ Premature death

National Bureau of Economic Research, the latter figure is even higher. These researchers found that obesity tacks on an extra $170 billion every year, or nearly 17 percent of the health-care expenditures in this country.[5]

As a physician, I'm particularly concerned about the toll that obesity takes on our health. Hippocrates said, "Corpulence is not only a disease itself, but the harbinger of others." Boy, was he right. Obesity is, without a doubt, the most serious medical problem confronting us today. It dramatically increases the risk of heart attack, stroke, high blood pressure, and other cardiovascular conditions. It is the primary factor in type 2 diabetes, which is a leading cause of kidney failure, lower-limb amputations, neuropathy, and blindness. Excess weight is also linked with rising rates of arthritis, liver disease, certain types of cancer, and more. And the consequences are more than physical. The psyche and ego suffer as well.

Dropping pounds in order to look and feel better is a perfectly acceptable goal. But I want you to understand that weight loss is about much more than a cute figure or a manly physique. It's a powerful remedy for preventing and treating a broad range of diseases. Let's look at the medical conditions most closely associated with obesity—and how the program outlined in this book has the potential to reverse many of today's most serious health challenges.

Diabetes + Obesity = Diabesity

As obesity rates have risen, so has the prevalence of diabetes. Nearly 26 million Americans, or more than 8 percent of the population, have diabetes, and another 79 million have "prediabetes," meaning that they're well on their way. The link between diabetes and obesity is so strong that it's led to the coining of a word: diabesity.

Let's examine why these two conditions are so closely intertwined. Type 2 diabetes, the kind that affects 95 percent of all people with diabetes, is caused by insulin resistance. Unlike those with type 1 diabetes, in which the beta cells in the pancreas are unable to produce enough insulin (the hormone that moves glucose from the blood into the cells), people with type 2 diabetes produce plenty of insulin. However, their cells are unresponsive, or resistant, to its signals, so glucose cannot enter the cells and blood sugar levels rise. The pancreas responds by secreting more insulin, resulting in elevated levels of both glucose *and* insulin.

BARIATRIC SURGERY: PROOF THAT WEIGHT LOSS WORKS

If you need proof that weight loss efforts are worth it, consider the studies on bariatric surgery. Bariatric procedures reduce the size of the stomach surgically (gastric bypass) or with the implantation of an adjustable band (Lap-Band), which radically restricts the amount of food that can be eaten at any given time.

The rapid and dramatic weight loss that bariatric surgery engenders dramatically improves diabetes and cardiovascular risk factors. Researchers at Johns Hopkins found that bariatric surgery eliminated diabetes in three-quarters of the patients who underwent the procedure—their diabetes literally disappeared! Within 6 months, the participants in this study were able to discontinue insulin and oral diabetes drugs, and over time, reduce the associated health-care costs from $10,000 to $1,800 per year.[6] Reversing obesity can also reverse cardiovascular disease. More than 9,000 morbidly obese patients were tracked for 5 years after their bariatric procedures, and at that time, their risk of heart attack, stroke, and death was slashed in half.[7]

I am not promoting bariatric surgery. It is a serious intervention for severely obese patients. Like all invasive procedures, it's fraught with risks and should be considered only as a last resort. However, the tremendous benefits that the patients in these studies reaped are proof that significant weight loss—preferably through lifestyle changes—is a U-turn on the road to disease and early death.

I want to make a quick comment about liposuction. Contrary to popular belief, liposuction is not a weight loss aid. It's a surgical intervention that removes excess fat deposits in order to reshape the body. Liposuction can certainly reduce saddlebags and love handles, but unless you keep your weight under control, the fat will return. In a 2011 study, a group of women who had liposuction on their thighs and/or lower abdomen were reevaluated 1 year after the procedure. Compared to a control group of women who did not have the procedure, there was no difference in terms of body fat. All the fat that had been suctioned out returned—but rather than on the thighs and the lower abdomen, it was redistributed in the upper abdomen, shoulders, and backs of the arms.[8]

High levels of insulin have a number of adverse effects, the most important in this discussion being weight gain. That's because insulin is also a fat-storage hormone. It ushers fatty acids into the muscles, the liver, and fat cells, and it shuts down the burning of fat for energy.

And if you're already overweight—as 90 percent of people with type 2 diabetes are—things go from bad to worse. Fat, especially the visceral adipose tissue in the abdominal area, is not the unsightly, inert mass we tend to think it is. Rather, it's a hotbed of metabolic activity. Visceral fat releases fatty acids that impair beta cell function. It is infiltrated by macrophages and other immune cells, which lead to chronic low-grade inflammation.[9] Excess fat also increases the production of, and decreases sensitivity to, leptin and other hormones that influence appetite, energy metabolism, and insulin sensitivity, resulting in reduced control over appetite and food intake.[10] Together, these obesity-induced abnormalities further increase insulin resistance and make blood sugar control and weight loss all the more challenging. (We will return to visceral fat in Chapter 7.)

Unfortunately, many of the usual treatments for diabetes do more harm than good. Physicians urge their diabetic patients to get their weight under control—and then prescribe drugs that make them heavier! In overweight people, insulin and most of the oral diabetes meds actually increase weight gain, making it more difficult to manage blood sugar and leading patients down a dark path toward painful, even life-threatening complications. I've had patients with type 2 diabetes who were morbidly obese *because* of their heavy insulin use. Once I discontinued the insulin and treated them with natural therapies—with no increase in their blood sugar levels—they were finally able to lose weight and control their diabetes. (To learn about these and other drugs that contribute to weight gain, turn to Chapter 8, "Removing Your Roadblocks.")

WEIGHT, WAISTS, AND DIABETES

In 1986, Harvard researchers launched the Health Professionals Follow-Up Study to examine the relationship between nutrition and disease. The study volunteers, a group of more than 50,000 male doctors, dentists, and other health-care professionals, have been checked every 2 years to the present, and the data mined from this long-term research project has led to more than 100 articles published in scientific journals.

One part of the study looked at the link between weight gain and diabetes, and found that for every kilogram (2.2 pounds) of additional weight, there was a 7.3 percent increase in the risk of diabetes. Furthermore, more than half of the men who developed diabetes had gained more than 15 pounds. Abdominal weight gain was the most perilous. Men whose waist size increased by more than 5½ inches had nearly double the risk of developing type 2 diabetes.[11]

There is a bright side. For most people dealing with type 2 diabetes, getting a handle on weight is all that it takes for blood sugar to normalize, complications to improve, and overall health to rebound.

The Healing Power of Weight Loss

Diet and exercise as treatments for diabetes and obesity require effort, but the payoff is worth it. Jason Davis, a Georgia resident and a subscriber to my monthly newsletter, *Health & Healing*, shared his story, which is a testament to the healing power of weight loss.

"A few years ago, at age 43, I was in the worst shape of my life. I am 6 feet 2, and I weighed 310 pounds, and the only exercise I got was mowing my yard. I insisted on going out for a fast-food lunch every day because I just 'had to get out of the office,' and those meals were usually 'supersized,' so I could get as much food as possible for my money.

"I already had hypertension and high cholesterol when a routine physical found a fasting blood sugar level of 160, and I was diagnosed with type 2 diabetes. Fortunately for me, my doctor gave me an ultimatum: I could either lose weight, or I would have to go on medication for the rest of my life. My wife was determined that I would not take any drugs. Following Dr. Whitaker's advice, I started exercising, and our whole family changed our lifestyle.

"It took time, but I lost more than 100 pounds and kept it off. I have never taken medication for diabetes, and my cholesterol

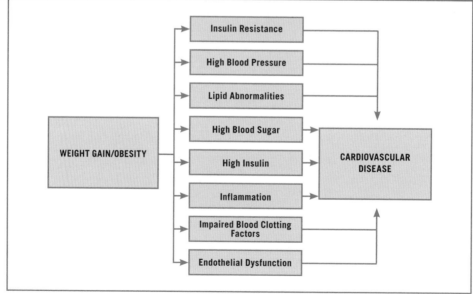

LINKS BETWEEN WEIGHT, METABOLIC SYNDROME, AND CARDIOVASCULAR DISEASE

and blood pressure are also under control. I now walk 4 miles 4 days a week, and climb Stone Mountain 2 days a week. I feel better than I have in years."

Granted, Jason's 100-pound weight loss is dramatic. However, losing just 5 to 10 percent of your body weight can also trigger tremendous improvements in type 2 diabetes and stave off complications and premature death.

Recounts Margaret D. of Laguna Niguel, California: "I had very good health until I turned 70. Then things started going bad. I didn't have a real doctor, so I would have to go to one of those walk-in clinics when I got a sore throat or something like that. I had to get myself a real doctor when my legs started hurting, and he diagnosed me with type 2 diabetes. My blood sugar level was over 300, and my blood pressure was elevated, too. I continued to see that doctor because he is a nice man, but then he started talking about having to amputate my toes and my feet and perform surgery for a hip condition. That is when I came to Dr. Whitaker's Wellness Institute.

"I am no longer the same woman. At Whitaker Wellness, they have miraculously taken care of practically all my problems. I only occasionally have stiffness in my hip, and some neuropathy and retinopathy. I've lost 25 pounds since I've been here without even trying and without being hungry, which is amazing because I was hungry all the time before. It is a wonderful thing to be able to fit into some of the clothes that I had put away in the back of the closet. I still have a few pounds and a little way to go as far as my cholesterol and blood pressure are concerned. Even old friends tell me that I haven't looked this way for ages, and I certainly haven't felt this way for ages. I have many things to be grateful for, and at the top of my list are this clinic and the people here."

MY APPROACH TO MEDICINE

I've been practicing medicine for more than 35 years, and the most gratifying aspect of being a doctor, bar none, is watching patients regain their health. That's what attracted me to the kind of medicine I practice today—we actually see patients get well.

Conventional medicine is great if you have a ruptured appendix or a broken bone. They fix you up and send you on your way. However, this same system does a very poor job when it comes to today's most pressing health challenges. If you're suffering with obesity, diabetes, hypertension, heart problems, arthritis, or another chronic, degenerative disorder, there's not even an expectation of finding an actual solution to your problem. Let's say you have high blood pressure, blood sugar, or cholesterol. Does your physician prescribe a medication for a month or two until your condition is "fixed," at which point you'll no longer need the drug? Of course not. The game plan is to "manage" you with increasing numbers of pharmaceuticals that you'll be taking for the rest of your life.

That is not wellness—and once I realized it nearly 4 decades ago, it changed my life and my career.

I QUESTIONED CONVENTIONAL MEDICINE

My medical training was essentially the same as any physician's. I graduated from Emory University Medical School in 1970, completed an internship at Grady Memorial Hospital in Atlanta, began a residency in San Francisco, and was looking forward to a career as an orthopedic surgeon. Then something happened. I was working in the emergency room one evening when a young woman came in. Aside from a sprained ankle, she was glowing with health and vitality, and when I commented on it, she credited her robust health in large part to nutritional supplements.

At that time, I didn't know much about nutrition—supplements or diet—because it wasn't something they taught us in medical school. But I was intrigued. This chance meeting led me first to Dr. Wilbur Currier in Pasadena, who turned me on to the extensive scientific medical literature on vitamins, minerals, and other nutrients. I was shocked at how much solid research was out there on the therapeutic value of nutrition. I had always assumed that if a therapy was safe, effective, and scientifically proven, it would be adopted by medicine, yet nutrition was inexplicably ignored.

That's about the time I began to question conventional medicine, with its dependency on prescription drugs, high-tech testing, invasive procedures—and the dismissal of most everything else. I left my residency and never looked back.

MY TRANSITION TO WELLNESS MEDICINE

In 1976, I worked as a staff physician at the Pritikin Longevity Center. Nathan Pritikin pioneered the use of a very low-fat, high-fiber, high-complex carbohydrate diet and exercise regimen for the treatment of diabetes and cardiovascular disease. Patients would come and stay at the facility for 4 weeks, eating a vegetarian diet ("rabbit food," as patients called it) and exercising by walking around like sentries guarding the property.

With diet and exercise—and these two therapies alone—patients lost weight. They got off their blood pressure meds, discontinued nitroglycerin, and stopped using insulin and oral diabetes drugs. They no longer needed them. In short, they got well. I knew this was the way I wanted to practice medicine. But I also knew that this couldn't be done within the usual confines of seeing the doctor, getting a prescription, and coming back in 2 months. Lifestyle changes require habit-breaking and habit-making, and that takes time and persistence. I wanted to create an environment where patients could come and stay for a while, learn how to eat right and exercise, optimize their nutritional status, and regain their health.

BIRTH AND GROWTH OF THE WHITAKER WELLNESS INSTITUTE

I opened the Whitaker Wellness Institute in 1979, a time when people were just beginning to look in earnest for alternatives in health care. I wrote a few books, including *Reversing Diabetes, Reversing Heart Disease,* and *Reversing Hypertension,* to get the word out about the downside of the conventional approach to these conditions and the nutritional and lifestyle therapies we use at the clinic. (*The Mini-Fast Diet* is my 14th book.)

(continued)

MY APPROACH TO MEDICINE *(cont.)*

In 1991, my monthly newsletter *Health & Healing* was launched. By this time the public was ready for provocative information about alternative medicine, and *Health & Healing* took off like a rocket, with circulation leaping to half a million subscribers in the first year. This increased exposure rapidly accelerated the growth of the clinic, and today the Whitaker Wellness Institute is the largest alternative medicine clinic in North America.

Over the years we have treated more than 50,000 patients, not with drugs and surgery but with the simple, inexpensive tools of diet, exercise, nutritional supplements, and safe, noninvasive therapies. We have sophisticated nutritional supplement protocols that we prescribe in place of medications for serious diseases. We use hyperbaric oxygen therapy to treat Parkinson's disease, heal wounds and infections, and facilitate recovery from trauma and stroke. We offer enhanced external counterpulsation (EECP) as an option to bypass and angioplasty for patients with cardiovascular disease. We provide relief from chronic pain with high-intensity laser treatment, infrared light, microcurrent, prolotherapy, acupuncture, chiropractic treatment, reflexology, and massage. We reduce heavy metal burden with chelation and boost nutritional status using intravenous (IV) vitamins and mineral protocols.

ADOPT LIFESTYLE CHANGES, LOSE WEIGHT, AND GET WELL

Despite this growth—which I never dreamed of 30-some years ago when I started the clinic—we have never lost sight of our original mission of treating serious diseases with

PUT THE BRAKES ON CARDIOVASCULAR DISEASE

Carrying around excess weight is also hard on your heart and circulatory system. This extra "baggage" and the metabolic abnormalities associated with it increase nearly every known risk factor for cardiovascular disease—beginning with endothelial dysfunction. The endothelium, a thin layer of cells lining the blood vessels,

lifestyle changes. Every patient who comes to the Whitaker Wellness Institute is pre-scribed a diet and exercise regimen and, if needed, a program for losing weight. Today, that need is greater than ever. A certain percentage of our population has always strug-gled with their weight, but when I started the clinic, obesity was relatively uncommon. Now, more people are obese than merely overweight, and rates of morbid obesity are rapidly increasing.

Many people are able to maintain their optimal weight on a healthy diet and exercise program. On the other hand, you need only look around you to know that many are not. That's why the Whitaker Wellness Institute's Back to Health Program is so effective. Patients come to Newport Beach, California, from all over the United States and Canada, stay in a nearby hotel, and for 1, 2, or 3 weeks, undergo therapies and immerse them-selves in a health-enhancing lifestyle. They also benefit from the company of like-minded individuals who are dissatisfied with conventional medicine's merry-go-round of drugs and surgery and are seeking to improve their health with safer, more natural means.

Many of the stories in this chapter—and throughout the book—are of people who spent some time with us learning or relearning healthy habits, experienced dramatic improvements, and left with the determination and belief that they could, and would, get well. The best part? They did! To learn more about the Whitaker Wellness Institute, go to www.whitakerwellness.com or call 800-488-1500.

plays a central role in cardiovascular health. Healthy endothelial cells discourage the formation of blood clots and the buildup of plaque in blood vessel walls and help keep inflammation and free radicals in check. It's easy to see why endothelial dysfunction has such widespread adverse effects.[12]

The vascular endothelium also releases nitric oxide, a signal-ing molecule that relaxes the arteries, improves circulation, and controls blood pressure. This is one reason, as weight increases or decreases, that blood pressure often follows suit. Hypertension is a common obesity-related condition. Epidemiological research suggests that at least 30 percent of hypertensive people are obese,[13] and hypertension, as you probably know, significantly increases the odds of suffering a stroke, a heart attack, heart failure, or an aneurysm.

Blood lipids also get out of kilter when you're heavy, particularly if you carry excess weight in the abdominal area. Levels of protective HDL cholesterol decline; triglycerides (fats circulating in the blood) go up; and concentrations of small, dense LDL cholesterol, which is particularly problematic, increase. In addition, obesity makes you more prone to developing blood clots, which can cause a heart attack or stroke when they lodge in a blood vessel. Obesity is also closely linked with elevated levels of highly sensitive C-reactive protein (hs-CRP), a marker of inflammation and an independent cardiovascular risk factor.

These factors combine to make obese individuals slow-moving targets for heart attacks, strokes, heart failure, and other serious cardiovascular conditions. Add insulin resistance and high blood sugar and insulin levels to the mix and you're a sitting duck. A Harvard research team looked at data from the Health Professionals Follow-Up Study mentioned on page 27 and the Nurses' Health Study, a "sister" project that focuses on women, and concluded that more than a third of all cases of cardiovascular disease in the US are associated with excess weight.[14]

No More Metabolic Syndrome

Again, the good news is that losing weight can reverse these underlying abnormalities and slash the risk of cardiovascular disease.

One of my patients, Ned, an electrical engineer and computer consultant from Oregon, had hypertension for almost 30 years. When he was first diagnosed, he was started on a blood pressure–lowering drug—the first of many, as it turned out. He couldn't tolerate the medication very well, so his doctor switched him to another, then another, until he'd tried just about every antihypertensive med on the market. Ned was sick and tired of feeling sick and tired, but he'd been told that drugs were his only option. So he came to see us at Whitaker Wellness.

We discovered that Ned, who had quite a bit of extra belly fat, had metabolic syndrome, which was contributing to his hypertension and increasing his risk of more serious problems down the road. We started him on a therapeutic diet, an exercise program,

DO YOU HAVE METABOLIC SYNDROME?

Metabolic syndrome is a cluster of risk factors that dramatically increase the odds of developing both type 2 diabetes and cardiovascular disease, and the underlying dysfunction is insulin resistance. Fueled by—and fueling—our epidemic of obesity, this syndrome is believed to affect 30 to 40 percent of Americans. If you have three or more of the following risk factors, you have metabolic syndrome; one or two, and you're headed in that direction. It's important to pay attention to these warning signs and get them under control before they turn into much bigger problems. The single most effective therapy? Weight loss.

- ✔ Abdominal obesity (waist circumference of more than 40 inches in men and 35 inches in women)
- ✔ Elevated blood pressure (130/85 or higher)
- ✔ High fasting blood glucose (100 mg/dL or above)
- ✔ Low HDL cholesterol (below 40 mg/dL in men and 50 mg/dL in women)
- ✔ Elevated triglycerides (150 mg/dL or higher)

and targeted nutritional supplements, and slowly weaned him off his drugs. Over the next year, as these lifestyle changes became second nature, he lost 30 pounds. A year and a half later, I ran into Ned at a conference in Las Vegas. He was fit, healthy, and feeling great, and his blood pressure averaged 125/75—without drugs.

Another patient, Billy C. from Rosamond, California, also had a long history of metabolic syndrome. He had been on blood pressure medication for 30 years, as well, and he had chest pain and shortness of breath. But when his cardiologist recommended bypass surgery, he decided to come to the Whitaker Wellness Institute instead. During his 3-week Back to Health Program, we treated his cardiovascular symptoms with natural therapies and weaned him off his prescription drugs. We also found that his blood sugar was a dangerously high 435—a clear-cut case of diabetes— and addressed that as well. He began exercising daily, modified his diet significantly, and started taking targeted nutritional supplements. By the time he left the clinic, his blood sugar readings were down to 89!

To date, Billy has lost 37 pounds and kept them off. He uses his treadmill and takes his supplements daily. He continues to maintain normal blood sugar and blood pressure levels and states, "You folks made my life 100 percent better."

MORE REASONS TO LOSE WEIGHT

Weight loss truly is one of the most powerful medical therapies. If it could be encapsulated, bottled, and sold by prescription, it would be the blockbuster of all blockbusters.

Let's look at a few other health problems closely tied to excess weight—and how they can be prevented or reversed by exercising, eating less, and getting your weight under control.

Stave Off Cancer

Obesity has been definitively linked with cancers of the colon, kidneys, esophagus, breasts, and endometrium, and there are tenuous associations with other malignancies. Extreme obesity is particularly problematic. A 16-year study conducted by the American Cancer Society found that morbid obesity increases the death rate from cancer by 62 percent in women and 52 percent in men.[15]

Everybody's scared of cancer because we're all aware of the horrendous side effects of conventional treatments such as chemotherapy and radiation. Most of us know someone who has been ravaged by these brutal therapies, only to succumb to cancer in the end. Furthermore, despite the trillions of dollars spent on the "war on cancer," death rates haven't declined all that much since the 1970s. That's why you need to do everything you can to reduce your risk—and that includes maintaining a normal weight.

Deliverance for Your Liver

The most common liver disease in the United States is not, as you may expect, hepatitis or alcoholic cirrhosis but nonalcoholic fatty liver disease (NAFLD). Affecting roughly one in four Americans, it isn't caused by alcohol or a virus but by abdominal obesity and insulin resistance. The hepatic portal vein, which drains blood from the gastrointestinal tract to the liver, lies in the abdominal cavity and—if you're overweight—smack in the middle of belly fat. To add fuel to the fire, insulin resistance impairs normal fat and glucose metabolism, resulting in an increased uptake and accumulation of fat in the liver.

NAFLD doesn't make you feel ill or jaundiced. The only real indication of this condition, besides abdominal obesity, is elevated liver enzymes, so most people don't even realize they have it.

However, NAFLD is a harbinger of future problems. Excess fat in the liver stimulates free-radical activity, which increases inflammation and, over time, damages hepatic cells. In some cases, NAFLD progresses to more serious nonalcoholic steatohepatitis (marked by inflammation), cirrhosis (scarring of the liver), and liver failure.

Studies suggest that NAFLD affects nearly 70 percent of people with type 2 diabetes and even more of those who are obese. But there is a cure: weight loss. Researchers at Saint Louis University found that when patients lost at least 9 percent of their body weight, they were able to reverse even advanced NAFLD. And exercise—independent of weight loss—also improved liver enzymes.[16]

Relieve the Adverse Effects of Sleep Apnea

Do you snore? Are you overweight? If you answered yes to either and especially both of these questions, odds are you have sleep apnea. When people with this condition sleep, the soft tissues in the back of the throat relax and close off the airway—they literally stop breathing. As oxygen levels plummet, they awake just enough to take a breath, and then the cycle repeats itself throughout the night.

Snoring is annoying to family members within earshot, but that's the least of it. Sleep involves several stages, and one of the deepest, most rejuvenating levels is rapid eye movement, or REM, sleep. During REM sleep, the brain unwinds and the muscles completely relax. It's also when the soft tissues in the throat collapse and apnea episodes occur. Although you may not be conscious of it, sleep apnea causes you to move out of REM sleep into lighter, less restorative sleep each time you're awakened to catch your

Barbara Hauth: "Motivated to Change and Improve My Health"

Barbara, who's from Pflugerville, Texas, was a svelte 5 feet 8 and 140 pounds when she started her family at age 22. She had three children in 5 years, and her body was just never able to bounce back between births. That was the beginning of a long struggle with weight that was compounded by life stresses, a hectic professional job, and raising a family. Her weight led to a host of medical problems, including type 2 diabetes, hypertension, high cholesterol, and sleep apnea. Here is Barbara's story.

"In the past I have lost 20 to 30 pounds on Weight Watchers and Nutrisystem. But I had considerably more to lose when I came to Whitaker Wellness in early 2011. Even though I knew what I needed to be eating (lean protein, more fruits and vegetables, more low-glycemic foods) for weight loss and my diabetes, the Whitaker Wellness Institute provided motivation, structure, education, and incentive to get back on track. When I returned home, I maintained the dietary changes and increased my exercise to 30 minutes a day, mostly swimming, walking, and dancing.

"The program is going well. Skipping breakfast has not been a big deal. Since I can drink water, tea, and coffee, I am not hungry before lunch. I watch my diet the rest of the day. My favorite foods on this program are salads, shrimp, salmon, tuna, chicken, and high-protein Greek yogurt. I enjoy low-glycemic fruits, and I take a number of nutritional supplements.

"Although I have not yet reached my target weight of 170, I know I am headed in the right direction. It is more than weight loss. The mini-fast and exercise in general help keep my blood sugar down. Plus, I feel so much better! I have told many others about the mini-fast. I also tell them that going to Dr. Whitaker's clinic is the best thing that I have done for myself! I am now, more than ever before, motivated to change and improve my health. I took back my life by going to the Whitaker Wellness Institute!"

breath. Consequently, it's virtually impossible to get enough restful sleep, even if you're clocking 8 hours a night.

Sleep apnea can wreak havoc on your health. In addition to causing fatigue and daytime sleepiness, it promotes inflammation, oxidative stress, hormonal imbalances, and insulin resistance. The fallout is significant: a two- to fivefold increased risk of stroke,

MINI-FAST, LIVE LONGER?

We've known since the 1930s that restricting calories reduces age-related disease and increases longevity. This has been demonstrated in every species from yeast and nematodes to rats and monkeys. Fruit flies, for example, live twice as long on a reduced-calorie diet, and mice live 35 to 50 percent longer. To date, it's the only proven intervention that consistently lengthens life span.

Calorie restriction switches on genes that encode a family of protective enzymes called sirtuins. Enzymes are proteins that catalyze (initiate and speed up) chemical reactions, and sirtuin enzymes play multiple roles in health and longevity. They facilitate DNA repair and maintain genome stability, protect against oxidative stress, and reduce inflammation. In lower organisms such as yeast, flies, and worms, a sirtuin called SIR2 is a key mediator, and its counterpart in mammals, SIRT1, has similar, though more complex, functions.

This is a very basic mechanism that evolved to ensure survival during times of food deprivation. Unfortunately, if you're overweight and overfed, these genes are rarely activated. Overeating and obesity also increase insulin levels, fuel inflammation, ramp up free radical production, and stimulate other physiological activities implicated in age-related disease. When you follow the mini-fast with exercise program, you will eat less and exercise more—activities that, to one degree or another, stimulate SIRT1 and tamp down inflammation, oxidative stress, and insulin overproduction. While research hasn't studied a mini-fast–longevity connection yet, based on what we do know, it's not a far-fetched concept that this plan could help you live longer.

hypertension, arrhythmia, and diabetes. It's also associated with heart failure, erectile problems, cancer, immune dysfunction, memory loss, and difficulty concentrating. Furthermore, it's both a cause *and* an effect of obesity. Excess weight sets the stage for sleep apnea—and sleep apnea leads to weight gain. It's a vicious circle, but it can be broken by weight loss.

If this discussion is hitting home for you, I strongly suggest that you talk to your doctor about getting tested for sleep apnea. At my clinic we screen patients with an overnight test that they can do in their homes. If the results are positive, they'll be prescribed treatment with an automatic positive airway pressure (APAP) or a continuous positive airway pressure (CPAP) machine. These devices, which are worn throughout the night, keep the airways open and put an end to sleep apnea episodes.

A Cure for Heartburn

Another health problem that's grown in tandem with our country's meteoric rise in obesity is gastroesophageal reflux disease (GERD). GERD is caused by a glitch in the esophageal sphincter, the ringlike muscle at the bottom of the esophagus that opens to let food and liquids into the stomach but otherwise remains closed to keep stomach contents from backing up into the esophagus. Abdominal obesity impairs function of this muscle and allows the reflux, or backward flow, of gastric acid to spill into the esophagus. Typical symptoms include heartburn and indigestion, but GERD may also cause chronic coughing, sore throat, hoarseness, and wheezing. It increases risk of esophageal cancer as well.

Far too many people with even minor heartburn are prescribed proton pump inhibitors (PPIs) such as Nexium, Prilosec, Prevacid, and Protonix. (Nexium is the leading brand-name drug sold in the US, raking in more than $5.6 billion in annual sales.) These drugs block the production of stomach acid and have a number of serious side effects, and one of which is weight gain—an average of 7.7 pounds over 2.2 years, according to one study.[17] Hands down, the safest and most effective therapy for GERD is weight loss. It alone is often enough to make GERD symptoms disappear for good.

F.W. from Texas reported, "I've had hypertension and gastroesophageal reflux disease (GERD) for several years, along with problems with my weight. Over the years I tried several drugs for both conditions, and when I went to Whitaker Wellness, I was taking Nexium for GERD and a blood pressure drug.

"Now I am off all meds, my blood pressure is within normal limits, and I have no GERD symptoms. I've lost my 'pudge' plus 21 pounds. My diet has improved dramatically. I used to crave sweets but don't now, and I do a lot of physical labor on my rental properties."

Similary, C.J.B. from Seal Beach, California, said, "My irritable bowel syndrome, acid reflux, and gas were so bad, I was afraid to walk into a store. When the drug my general practitioner put me on didn't help, he said, 'I don't know what to do for you.' So I went to the Whitaker Wellness Institute. Now here I am, 77 years young and 18 pounds lighter, and I feel like a young chick again. I have nothing but praise for your clinic."

Save Your Joints

About 50 million American adults have been diagnosed with osteoarthritis, a degeneration of the cartilage that cushions the joints, and this number is expected to grow by about a million per year over the next 2 decades. A driving force behind this increase is obesity.[18] One in three obese women and one in four obese men have arthritis, as do more than half of those considered to be morbidly obese. When you think about it, this comes as no surprise.

Carting around an extra 20, 30, or 40 pounds does a number on your joints; and your hips, ankles, and knees—the most common sites of osteoarthritis—bear the brunt of it.

Losing weight takes stress off your joints, slows cartilage erosion, and reduces the likelihood of requiring a knee or hip replacement in the future. Younger people may have a hard time grasping the gravity of this, but you need to realize that if you're seriously overweight, this degenerative process has already begun. Your best bet is to take action now.

ONE PLAN, MANY BENEFITS

To sum up, obesity's adverse effects impact virtually every organ system in the body. In addition to those discussed above, kidney and gallbladder disease, asthma and gout, infertility and urinary incontinence, and dementia and Alzheimer's disease are also linked with excess weight. I don't want to paint too dark a picture, but you must understand that being overweight is not merely a cosmetic issue. We as a country—and you as an individual—can no longer afford to overlook the personal, social, economic, and medical burdens of obesity. It's time to get real about weight loss. In the next chapter, I'll tell you how.

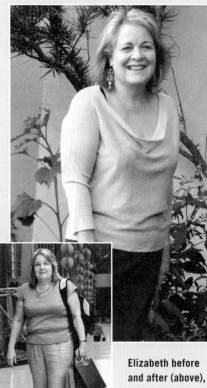

Elizabeth before and after (above), 25 pounds lighter.

Elizabeth Billups: "The Best Birthday Present I Could Have Ever Given Myself"

"I started the mini-fast in April 2010, when I first went to the Whitaker Wellness Institute. At that time I was overweight and had uncontrolled diabetes. I was mad at first when my doctor there wanted me to try it. I hadn't come to the clinic to learn to fast; I had come to learn to eat properly. I had always been told that people with blood sugar problems need to eat all day long. I also was worried that I would be faint or weak trying to exercise on an empty stomach. And like most everyone else, I 'knew' that breakfast was the most important meal of the day.

"I was wrong on all counts. The mini-fast is brilliant! I have been on it for over a year now and lost about 25 pounds—and I no longer have diabetes.

"When I started on this program, I was in bad shape. I had been diagnosed with diabetes with a blood sugar so high that the lab questioned whether or not I had been fasting. My doctor back home in Santa Fe put a lot of pressure on me to start taking a drug right then and there. However, my dad, uncle, and other family members had diabetes and had been on numerous meds, including insulin, yet still had serious complications. I was convinced I could do this on my own.

"I tried other diets, but it was always a struggle, and I just couldn't stick with them. After a while, the thought of taking a pill and being able to eat whatever

I wanted started to sound good. So I sought out another physician, who was more than willing to write a prescription. He also wanted to put me on a blood pressure medication, even though my blood pressure was low/normal, because, as he said, 'most diabetics get hypertension.' That did it. I walked out, went home, and called Whitaker Wellness.

"When I arrived, my diabetes was out of control. My blood sugar was 300 and my hemoglobin A1C was 12.8 [normal is 4 to 6 percent]. My doctor put me on the mini-fast with exercise program, lots of nutritional supplements, and bioidentical hormones (thyroid, estrogen, progesterone). During my 2-week stay, I attended the lectures and saw the nutritionist and learned that the 'healthy' carbohydrates I had been eating weren't so healthy after all. I quickly got used to eating the lean protein, vegetables, and low-glycemic foods served at the clinic. I also underwent hyperbaric oxygen therapy and other treatments that did wonders for the neuropathy in my feet and chronic pain in my neck.

"After I returned home, I was a little nervous about whether or not I would be able to do it on my own. I've never considered myself to be someone who has a lot of discipline, but I find this program is very easy to stay on. Basically, I haven't had breakfast in over a year. On my day off, I might have a late breakfast around 10:30 or so, but I've adjusted very well. The food at the clinic was fantastic, and I was able to replicate it at home. I've always been a good exerciser, but once I started on the mini-fast, everything began falling into place.

"Within 6 months, my blood sugar and A1C were completely normal. Based on these numbers, I'm considered to be a nondiabetic at this point. However, I know I'll always have that tendency, and I'm committed to maintaining control of my health. Going to the Whitaker Wellness Institute and learning about the mini-fast was the best thing I have ever done. I celebrated my 59th birthday at the clinic, and it was the best birthday present I could have ever given myself. The weight I've lost has stayed off. I look and feel better than I have in years, and because of my enthusiasm, five people in Santa Fe are now also on the mini-fast."

CHAPTER 3

WHY THE MINI-FAST WITH EXERCISE WORKS

From the standpoint of promoting leanness, exercise is of most value if oxidation [burning] of stored fat is maximized during and following the exercise sessions. . . . This protocol, combining elements of exercise training, fasting, and low-fat eating, is both sustainable and healthful, and in reasonably compliant subjects may have considerable potential for promoting and maintaining leanness and insulin sensitivity.

—BAHADORI, B., MCCARTY, M.F., ET AL., "A 'MINI-FAST WITH EXERCISE' PROTOCOL FOR FAT LOSS"[1]

The calories-in, calories-out model of weight loss is obviously oversimplistic. There's an expectation that if you do a certain amount of exercise or cut a particular number of calories, you'll lose weight. But as you may have experienced firsthand, A plus B doesn't always equal C. You take the time and effort to exercise and suffer the deprivation of following a special diet, but you don't get the results you hoped for.

What makes the mini-fast with exercise different and far more effective than other regimens is the *timing.* This is a concept so simple, so logical, and—once you "get it"—so obvious that it's like discovering that the missing eyeglasses you've been searching for are sitting right on your nose.

In order to appreciate the power of this program, you need to understand how your body uses and stores energy. Most important, you need to learn how to redirect energy creation and utilization toward burning fat, which is the ultimate goal in weight loss.

ENERGY 101

Carbohydrates are the body's preferred source of energy. Whether they're small, simple sugar molecules like sucrose and fructose or long-chain starches, carbohydrates are broken down in the digestive process into glucose, which is the body's primary fuel. As glucose enters the bloodstream, it signals the pancreas to secrete insulin, the hormone that lets glucose and other nutrients enter the cells. Once taken up, glucose is metabolized along with oxygen in the mitochondria, the cells' "power stations," to produce ATP, the basic unit of energy that runs your brain, muscles, and other physiological functions. Fats and proteins can also be burned for energy, but their conversion into a usable form is more complex, and as a fuel source, they take a backseat to glucose. Whenever carbohydrates are present, they are used first.

Important as carbohydrates are, the body has a very limited capacity for storing them. Some glucose is converted into glycogen, the storage form of carbohydrates that is akin to starch in plants, and stockpiled in the liver and the muscles. Excess glucose can be converted into fat for long-term storage in adipose, or fat, cells. This conversion, called de novo lipogenesis, occurs to a meaningful extent only when people gorge themselves, eating far more carbs than necessary and filling their glycogen stores until they practically burst (which a lot of us do). Blood glucose and insulin levels then taper off until you eat again. Several hours after eating, and during the night, glycogen is slowly broken down and converted back into glucose to fuel your basic biological processes.

Now let's look at fat. When you eat dietary fats, they are absorbed from the digestive tract, processed in the liver, and released into the bloodstream, primarily in the form of triglycerides. Adipose cells readily take up triglycerides and store them until they're needed for energy. The more fat you eat, the more you store. This means that—quite literally—the fat you eat is the fat you wear on your belly and hips. If you eat a lot of red meat and eggs, your adipose cells contain an abundance of saturated fats; if your diet leans more toward monounsaturated olive oil and omega-3–rich salmon, these will be the predominant fatty acids in your adipose tissue.

Unlike the storage of carbohydrates, the body's capacity for fat storage is huge, even in people who are thin. A fit, athletic man's total body weight comprises 6 to 13 percent fat, and an athletic woman's is in the 14 to 20 percent range. A man with a decent body composition (15 percent fat) would have 30 pounds of stored fat, while the "average" American male lugs around more than 50 pounds of fat. For normal-weight women, we're talking 35 to 40 pounds of fat, to more than 60 pounds of it for those who are overweight.

Some of that fat is "essential," meaning that it's required to cushion the organs, sheathe the nerves, maintain cellular structure, and

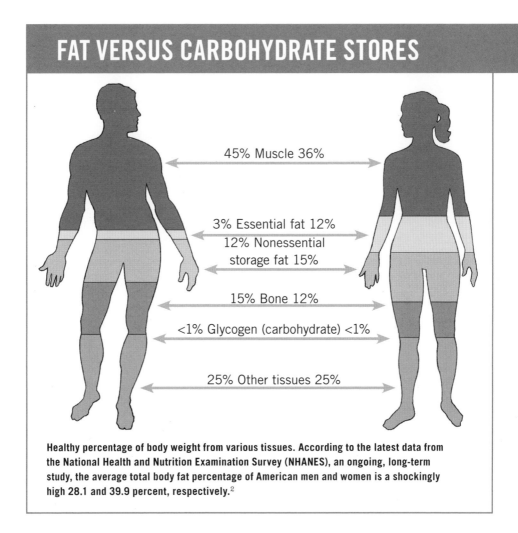

FAT VERSUS CARBOHYDRATE STORES

45% Muscle 36%

3% Essential fat 12%

12% Nonessential
storage fat 15%

15% Bone 12%

<1% Glycogen (carbohydrate) <1%

25% Other tissues 25%

Healthy percentage of body weight from various tissues. According to the latest data from the National Health and Nutrition Examination Survey (NHANES), an ongoing, long-term study, the average total body fat percentage of American men and women is a shockingly high 28.1 and 39.9 percent, respectively.[2]

perform myriad other functions that keep you alive. Women's essential fat is higher than men's because extra fat is needed in the breasts, pelvis, hips, and thighs to carry out normal reproductive functions. On the other hand, nonessential fat—as the name suggests—you can do without. It's the unsightly stuff protruding from your abdomen, thighs, buttocks, and elsewhere. The only way to get rid of this fat is to coax it out of adipose cells and use it for energy.

WHAT IS KETOSIS?

Fat is an excellent source of energy, but it is not as "green" as glucose. When the body burns fat, it makes by-products: small carbon fragments called ketones. Ketosis is the presence of elevated levels of ketones in the blood. In essence, it's a marker of fat burning.

Ketones are also used for energy. In fact, they make very efficient fuel, especially for the heart muscle. And in the absence of glucose, they're vital for the brain, which cannot use fat directly for energy. A ketogenic diet—very high in fat with almost no carbohydrates, which results in robust levels of ketones—is a proven therapy for seizure disorders. Ketones are also being researched as a promising treatment for Alzheimer's disease and other neurodegenerative disorders.

When ketones accumulate in the blood faster than they can be used, some are expelled from the body via the urine and the lungs. You may be familiar with the sweet, fruity smell on the breath associated with ketosis—it's caused by exhaling a ketone called acetone. Expelling ketones is like putting logs on the fire, allowing them to burn three-quarters of the way down, then discarding the still-burning logs and replacing them with new ones. Obviously, you'll burn up more wood this way. Likewise, when you're burning fat and throwing off ketones, you're depleting your fat stores. Ketosis also curbs appetite,

Although the body is primed to metabolize carbohydrates for energy, it seamlessly changes over to its backup source when glucose and glycogen stores are unavailable. Like a long-haul trucker switching over to a supplemental gas tank, the body begins to burn fat.

Fat burning is the payoff for the ancient biological drive we discussed in the first chapter: to overeat high-calorie foods whenever they're available. This instinct is what kept our distant ancestors going in times of scarcity—between successful hunts, for example, and during the cold season, when plant foods were harder to come by.

another evolutionary adaptation that makes going without food more tolerable. You're simply not as hungry when you're in this mode, and this makes skipping a meal much easier that you might expect.

There is a widespread myth that ketosis is dangerous. An exceptionally high blood level of ketones—an acidic condition called ketoacidosis—is indeed dangerous and may cause organ damage and death. However, this is rare and is seen primarily in individuals with uncontrolled type 1 diabetes. The degree of ketosis that occurs while on a low-carbohydrate diet or the mini-fast with exercise program is a natural state and, as such, is inherently safe. Do not forget that our hunter-gatherer ancestors spent extended periods in ketosis.

In summary, the mini-fast with exercise is all about fat burning. Ketosis is a by-product of fat burning and is therefore an obvious goal. But it should not be your primary focus. This program does not require that you strictly avoid carbohydrates, eat lots of fat, or urinate on Ketostix or other ketone test strips to make sure that you're in ketosis. Just concentrate on three steps—skip breakfast, do morning exercise, and eat sensibly—and the loss of pounds, inches, and clothing sizes is sure to follow. (Not a morning person? As you'll see in Chapter 5, the mini-fast with exercise can be modified to fit any schedule.)

For better *and* for worse, this natural mechanism is hardly ever triggered in most of us these days. There's a clear upside to this. It means that, for the majority of people in developed countries, the specter of starvation is no longer a threat. We complain about rising costs, but we are indeed fortunate to be living in a time and place where, relatively speaking, affordable food is readily accessible. From a historical perspective, this is exceedingly rare, and even to this day, millions of people worldwide die of starvation every year.

The downside is that a lot of us are fat. Our instincts compel us to overeat in order to stockpile energy for leaner times, yet those times never come. We continually deposit fat but never withdraw it. Furthermore, we "graze" all day, which keeps our insulin levels up and our ability to burn fat down. The environment we find ourselves in today has essentially eliminated nature's checks and balances. Therefore, you must create an effective strategy for burning fat. Your options are to reduce calories rather dramatically and exercise quite intensely—or to follow the program outlined in the Mini-Fast Diet, which combines the two in a moderate, scientifically proven way to accelerate fat burning, blunt hunger, reduce weight, and improve overall health.

CUT CALORIES WITH RELATIVE EASE

Calorie reduction alone facilitates weight loss, but as everyone knows, it's awfully difficult to keep up for very long. The usual recommendations on a calorie-restricted diet—1,800 calories per day for men and 1,200 for women—require taking quite a chunk out of the average US daily allotment of about 2,500 calories for men and 1,800 for women.[3] The 600 to 700 calories you would have to eliminate are one-third to one-fourth of your entire daily intake!

Most people try to accomplish this by consuming smaller portions and limiting second helpings. They replace high-calorie foods with lower-calorie alternatives or eliminate a specific item or category such as desserts, fast foods, fat, or carbohydrates. Some go the meal-replacement route, swapping out regular food for energy bars, shakes, or prepared meals. Others adhere to specific diets and meal plans or get help from a support group like Weight Watchers.

The stumbling block in calorie restriction is appetite. Although we use the terms interchangeably, appetite is not the same thing as hunger. Hunger is a physiological need for food, a physical sensation that drives us to eat. Orchestrated by an elaborate network of hormones, neurotransmitters, and other messenger molecules, hunger lets us know when we need to eat and when to stop. Appetite also compels us to eat, but it's more of a desire than a physiological need. We don't have to be hungry, i.e., require sustenance, in order to want a hamburger or a muffin. The mere sight, smell, or thought of food can compel us to eat. And we all know how difficult it is to turn down a favorite food when it's right in front of us. Think of it like this: When you're hungry, you eat a sandwich, but it's appetite that drives you to eat another one because the first one tasted so darn good.

There are a few tricks for dampening appetite, which we'll discuss in greater detail in subsequent chapters. They include eating bulky, fiber-rich, highly satiating foods; having protein with every meal and snack; eliminating high-glycemic carbohydrates that lead to blood sugar swings and food cravings; and taking appetite-suppressing nutritional supplements. Drastically reducing carbohydrates, the principle behind the Atkins diet, also curbs appetite (for the same reason the mini-fast does). But most folks miss their carbs and find it hard to stick with this approach over the long term.

Far easier than wrestling with appetite and temptation, making uncomfortable food choices, and counting calories all day long is simply eliminating a meal: mini-fasting. I know this goes against both the popular notion that you have to eat three meals a day and the advice commonly given to dieters to eat even more often, with small snacks between meals. Plus, it flies in the face of the commandment that breakfast is the most important meal of the day. (Breakfast is also the easiest meal to skip, as we'll discuss in Chapter 4, Why Breakfast *Isn't* the Most Important Meal of the Day.)

(continued on page 56)

FASTING: THE ULTIMATE WEIGHT LOSS AND HEALTH RESTORATION PROGRAM

I once saw a T-shirt that said "Ask me how to lose weight" on the front and "Stop eating" on the back. It's meant to be funny, but not eating—fasting—is the ultimate weight loss program.

Humans have been fasting since time immemorial. Abstaining from food has long been considered a spiritual practice and continues to be a tenet of all of the world's major religions. Jesus fasted for 40 days and 40 nights, and Buddha meditated for 49 days without eating or drinking. Jews fast on Yom Kippur, and Muslims take no food or water from sunup to sundown during the month of Ramadan. However, I'm not here to discuss the religious ramifications of fasting but its profound effects on health.

Fasting is a unique and very powerful therapy. In addition to promoting weight loss, it rapidly rids the body of excess sodium and fluids, eliminates edema, and lowers blood pressure.[4] It improves insulin sensitivity and virtually every aspect of metabolic syndrome. By mobilizing and eliminating stored toxins, fasting is a great detoxification regimen. It gives the gastrointestinal tract a chance to repair itself, which often leads to dramatic improvements not only in chronic digestive problems but also in allergies and autoimmune diseases. Furthermore, fasting activates SIRT1 genes that reduce inflammation and oxidative stress and increase cell survival—and actually improve longevity.

ENDURING BENEFITS OF FASTING

That's all well and good, but what about after the fast ends? Studies indicate that benefits are enduring. Alan Goldhamer, DC, is founder and director of TrueNorth, a clinic in Santa Rosa, California, that specializes in medically supervised fasting. For the past 25 years, TrueNorth has helped more than 7,000 patients overcome obesity, hypertension, diabetes, and other health challenges with 5- to 40-day fasts. What he and others have found is that fasting seems to reset metabolism, much like rebooting resets your computer, and makes it run better. Taking a break from eating interrupts the vicious circles that lock into place disorders such as hypertension and diabetes. When people with these problems undergo fasts that average 7 to 10 days, followed by the adoption of a healthy lifestyle and accompanied by appropriate weight loss, they often succeed in quickly reversing these conditions.[5]

Dr. Goldhamer and his colleagues reported on 174 of their hypertensive patients who were treated with fasting. At the conclusion of the fasts, 90 percent had achieved normal blood pressure, with average reductions of 37/13 mm Hg, and all antihypertensive medications had been discontinued. These patients were then gradually started on a plant-based, whole-food diet low in salt and high in potassium—the kind of diet that prevents hypertension in the first place—and sent home with instructions to stay on this healthy plan. A number of the participants were tracked for an average of 27 weeks after leaving the clinic, and their mean blood pressure remained a perfectly healthy 123/77.[6]

Fasting also has a lasting effect on diabetes. When I was a medical student at Emory University and an intern at Grady Memorial Hospital in Atlanta, John K. Davidson, MD, PhD, was a professor at the university and the director of the hospital's diabetes unit. This very conventional physician used fasting as a treatment for diabetes. In his popular medical textbook, he described how a 7-day fast as the initial treatment for obese patients with type 2 diabetes resulted in predictable improvements in blood sugar, weight, and blood pressure—and not only during the fast. These patients transitioned to low- to moderate-calorie diets, and over the next 5 to 7 months, they gradually got down to their ideal weight and gained control of their blood sugar without the use of insulin or oral diabetes drugs.[7]

A SAFE, EFFECTIVE THERAPY

I want to dispel the common yet absolutely erroneous idea that fasting is dangerous. This belief, which has been accepted by Western medicine for more than a century, has no scientific basis whatsoever, but somehow it has taken hold. The following story, from Dr. Goldhamer's book *The Pleasure Trap,* taken from the 1877 annals of medical history, is a great example of fasting's safety and therapeutic value.

(continued)

FASTING: THE ULTIMATE WEIGHT LOSS AND HEALTH RESTORATION PROGRAM (*cont.*)

Henry Tanner was a physician who suffered from such excruciating rheumatism, asthma, and poor sleep that he felt life wasn't worth living and decided to end it all. The method of demise he settled on was to starve himself to death, as in those days, everybody "knew" that going 10 days without food would be fatal. He shut himself up in his house, drank water but refused all food, and waited to die. A few days into his fast, unexpected things began to happen. His pain dramatically decreased, and for the first time in years, he began to sleep like a baby. By day 11, he was feeling "as well as in my youthful days." He continued to fast for 31 days, and during that time, all of his symptoms abated. When he shared his experience, his fellow physicians ridiculed him and called his fasting story a fraud. But Dr. Tanner had the last laugh. He lived to the ripe old age of 90 pain free and in excellent health.[8]

My final comments on this subject: Extended fasting is much easier for anyone to do in a supportive setting. I would not recommend that anyone with a serious health problem undergo a prolonged fast without medical supervision. Fasters, even short-termers, need to drink a lot of water, relax, and take it easy, and to break the fast with fresh vegetable and fruit juices, followed by the gradual introduction of whole, natural, unprocessed foods. To learn more about medically supervised fasting at TrueNorth, visit www.healthpromoting .com or call 707-586-5555.

Obviously, if you miss one meal a day, you're making a significant dent in your overall food intake. Depending on what you usually eat, that meal could contain the 25 to 33 percent of the calories most people need to give up in order to lose weight. If skipping breakfast sounds like torture, I urge you to just try it—it really isn't all that tough. Because you won't be eating the usual high-carb foods, you won't have the blood sugar crashes that often lead to midmorning food cravings. I'm not saying that forgoing one meal is sufficient to promote significant weight loss. It is possible that you'll end up feeling hungrier and eating more later in the day than you would have otherwise. But what if there was a way to ensure that you wouldn't be hungry—and that more of your energy needs would be met by burning stored fat? That's where exercise comes in.

EXERCISE WHEN IT REALLY COUNTS

Exercise long enough and hard enough and you'll burn fat. However, you have to do a heck of a lot of physical activity to significantly reduce your weight. As I said in the first chapter, exercise alone is not an effective weight loss strategy. But that's because little consideration is given to the context and timing in which it's done.

The mini-fast with exercise takes advantage of the natural fast you undertake every night. Let's say that you finish dinner at 8:00 p.m. By the time you get up at 6:00 or 7:00 the next morning, you will have fasted for 10 to 11 hours. At that point, your body is beginning to deplete the glycogen that was deposited in your liver and muscles from the carbohydrates you ate at your evening meal. Even if you didn't exercise but put off breakfast and continued to fast until noon, you would be whittling down your glycogen stores and beginning to rely on fat for energy. But when you exercise in the morning—while still in this fasting state—you rev up your engine. You blow through your remaining glycogen and go straight into burning fat. And until you eat, you will remain in that fat-burning state. As you can see, omitting breakfast *and* exercising does much more than reducing a meal's worth of calories or exercising alone.

Now let's say that you eat before working out, even if it's something small like a granola bar or a glass of juice. You will do a great job of burning the carbohydrates you just ingested for energy, but you will not burn fat. Another common scenario is to eat right after exercising. This too turns off the fat burning that exercise may have triggered. It stops it right in its tracks!

The solution? Work out *during* the morning mini-fast and wait until noon to eat, and you will burn off stored fat for hours. Provided that the food you eat the rest of the day is relatively low in fat and that you don't go overboard on calories, you will not replace the fat stores you're depleting—and you'll be on the road to optimal weight and robust health.

SCIENTIFIC SUPPORT FOR THE PROGRAM

I first learned about the mini-fast with exercise from Mark McCarty, a prolific writer and researcher whom I've known and worked with for years. Mark completed 3 years of medical school before deciding that he was more interested in nutrition than in treating patients. So he focused his efforts on nutritional research, and over the past 25 years, he has had more than 240 scientific papers published in biomedical journals.

Years ago, Mark was in Tokyo for an international scientific conference when he was struck by a sudden observation: There were no fat people. He saw, literally, only one overweight Japanese man during his entire visit. Upon his return to the States, however, every other person he ran into was either overweight or downright obese. Haunted by this stark contrast, he delved into the medical literature and found that the traditional Japanese diet is exceptionally low in fat, about 10 percent of daily calories, and high in carbohydrates, especially rice. He also learned that humans have a limited capacity to convert dietary carbohydrate to fat. The con-clusion was clear—if you eat a diet very low in fat and don't stuff yourself on carbohydrates beyond your calorie requirements, you are unlikely to ever get fat. The effortless leanness of the Japa-nese at that time was living proof. (While the obesity rate in Japan is on the rise, it's still less than 5 percent, as compared with 34 percent in the United States.)

Mark recognized that simply adopting a low-fat diet wouldn't necessarily *reverse* obesity in people who are already heavy. Dietary carbohydrate may not be efficiently converted to body fat unless it's eaten in excess. However, eating even modest amounts increases blood glucose and insulin levels, which block the body's burning of stored fat and thus prevent weight loss.[9] Therefore, to promote weight loss, a low-fat, moderate-calorie diet would be most effective combined with a strategy to boost fat burning, such as exercise—provided that the exercise was conducted in a way to selectively burn stored fat. This train of thought led him to the concept of the "mini-fast with exercise."

In 1995, he wrote a paper titled "Optimizing Exercise for Fat Loss," in which he put forth the theory that, from the standpoint of promoting fat loss, prolonged moderate-intensity exercise is most effective when done in the morning after fasting overnight, especially if no calories are ingested for several hours following exercise. If subsequent meals are relatively low in fat, the fat burned off during and after exercise won't be replaced, leading to a loss of body fat that, over weeks and months, could be quite significant. As the body becomes leaner, the amount of fat burned with exercise will decline until it equals the amount of fat supplied by the low-fat diet, and weight will equilibrate. This new, leaner equilibrium can be maintained as long as the mini-fast with exer-cise strategy is continued. And there is no reason that anyone will-ing to exercise regularly couldn't keep this up indefinitely.[10]

Mark is his own best study subject. On this protocol, he lost two-thirds of his body fat and was so pleased with the results that he has followed this program, along with a low-fat vegan diet and a comprehensive nutritional supplement program, for nearly 15 years. He's in excellent health and has a very lean body composition of 5 percent fat. He shared these ideas with Austrian physician Babak Bahadori, MD, who adapted them into a seven-step program for weight control, which has achieved outstanding results for his patients and others who have followed his regimen. At the Whitaker Wellness Institute, the nation's largest alternative medicine clinic, the mini-fast with exercise is the primary weight loss strategy, prescribed by physicians and enthusiastically embraced by patients who have had greater, more lasting success than with any other approach.

In addition to this clinical experience, a number of scientific studies have evaluated the basic concepts of the program—including a very impressive 12-week clinical trial of the mini-fast with exercise. Here's a brief overview of the research.

Exercising before Breakfast Prevents Weight Gain

Belgian researchers interested in whether the timing of exercise in relation to eating had differing effects on health and weight enrolled active, healthy young men in a 6-week study. During the trial period, the participants were required to eat a really bad diet. They consumed a third more calories than they were accustomed to, and 50 percent of their calories were from fat. It was in effect a recipe for weight gain. The men were then divided into three groups:

♦ Group one ran and/or cycled at a good clip for 60 to 90 minutes four mornings a week before breakfast. The only thing they were allowed to consume prior to and during exercise was water.

- Group two had an identical intense exercise protocol, but the men worked out after eating a hearty, carbohydrate-dense meal. They were also given carbohydrate-containing beverages to drink during exercise.

- Group three served as the control group. These men were instructed to refrain from exercising for the study's duration and to simply eat the lousy diet.

As expected, the control group of overeating, nonexercising men gained weight, about a pound a week, for a total gain of a little more than 6 pounds on average. They also had significant fatty deposits in their muscles and elsewhere and developed insulin resistance, which, as we discussed in the previous chapter, is the underlying cause of metabolic syndrome. Just 6 weeks of sitting around and gorging on fatty foods started these fit young men down the road toward obesity and poor health.

What was really interesting about this study is that group two, the men who exercised after eating breakfast, also gained weight, about 3 pounds. They too had impaired insulin sensitivity and increased fat stores in their muscles. Those in group one, however, who exercised in a fasting state before breakfast, did not gain weight or store fat. They did not develop insulin resistance. Remember, these men also ate an unhealthy, high-calorie, high-fat diet. The only difference was that because they exercised before eating—a primary principle of the mini-fast with exercise—they burned fat far more efficiently.[11]

Modest Calorie Restriction plus Exercise

Another clinical trial was conducted by researchers who wanted to see if the disease-preventing, health-enhancing, life span–extending effects of calorie restriction—which, as we discussed in Chapter 2, are clearly evident in other species—work in humans. Now, studying calorie restriction in humans is very, very difficult. People aren't compliant when it comes to reducing their food intake. ("Calorie restriction," as the old joke goes, "may not actually make you live longer, but it sure feels that way.")

To that end, the National Institute on Aging sponsored a multicenter study called Comprehensive Assessment of the Long-Term Effects of Reducing Intake of Energy (CALERIE). The institute recruited highly motivated and organized people who were willing to commit to 2 years of calorie restriction, scrupulous documentation of their diets and exercise, and frequent reevaluation. Several papers have come out of this study, including one from the Pennington Biomedical Research Center, in Baton Rouge, Louisiana, that sheds light on the benefits of the mini-fast with exercise program. This 6-month study involved healthy but overweight men and women who were divided into three groups:

- Group one followed a calorie-restricted diet, a 25 percent reduction in total calories eaten.

- Group two restricted calories by 12.5 percent *and* increased their caloric expenditure by 12.5 percent via a boost in exercise.

- Group three was the control group, and made no changes to their diets or exercise.

Over the 6 months, the control group lost the least amount of weight, an average of 1.4 pounds plus 1.4 percent of their body fat. No surprise there. But what I found fascinating about this study is that the men and women in the other two groups lost similar amounts of weight: about 18 pounds and 5.4 to 6 percent of their fat mass. This means that in this carefully controlled group, significant calorie reduction (25 percent fewer calories) and moderate reduction (12.5 percent fewer) plus moderate exercise stimulated significant weight and fat loss. Both groups also had improvements in insulin sensitivity, increased mitochondrial biogenesis (the creation of new mitochondria, the cells' energy producers, in the muscles), reduced DNA damage, decreased oxidative stress, and turned-on SIRT1 ("antiaging") gene expression.[12]

MINI-FAST FINALLY GOT RID OF STUBBORN BELLY FAT

Sue Anderson is one of our most senior and valued members of the Whitaker Wellness team. If you'd seen her before she started on the mini-fast with exercise program, you wouldn't have thought she had a weight problem. That's because she has never let her weight get completely out of control. Nevertheless, she's always had to work at it, and is a lifetime member of Weight Watchers. She had one reason and one reason only for trying the mini-fast with exercise program: to lose her "belly fat," which just wouldn't budge.

Mission accomplished! Sue lost 8 pounds, dropping from 131 to 123—but nearly 7 pounds of that was fat, and her waist circumference shrank by 4½ inches!

When I talked to Sue about the program, she said: "I take a 40-minute walk every morning, and I also do Jazzercise three or four times a week. As far as breakfast goes, I really don't miss it, and I try to eat nutritious meals the rest of the day. Sometimes I fall off the wagon, but all this exercise allows me to get by with occasional discretions. I continue to regularly weigh in at Weight Watchers because this keeps me on track. However, I also plan to stay on the mini-fast and exercise in the morning. I can tell you from personal experience that this program really does turn on fat burning. No matter how much I exercised and how little I ate, I couldn't get rid of those last few stubborn pounds around my midsection—until I started on the mini-fast with exercise."

I concluded my interview with Sue by asking how she managed to fit in exercise in the mornings, because I know she arrives at work early. She said, "Easy. I just get up at 4:30 every day."

The take-home message is that modest calorie restriction (a 12.5 percent cut isn't Draconian) and moderate exercise—in other words, the mini-fast with exercise—is an excellent strategy for weight reduction and better health.

Mini-Fast with Exercise Clinical Trial

The mini-fast with exercise itself was evaluated in a 2009 clinical trial. This 12-week study involved 27 overweight volunteers— 17 women and 10 men—weighing an average of 199 pounds, with a BMI of 32.2 (30 and above is considered obese), a waist circumference of 42.6 inches, and fasting insulin of 13.2 IU/mL (a level indicative of insulin resistance). They were instructed to engage in some form of aerobic exercise for 45 minutes, performed during a 12- to 14-hour mini-fasting period, for a minimum of 3 to 5 days a week. There were no dietary restrictions, but the participants were encouraged to eat a low-fat, low-glycemic, high-fiber diet.

Twelve weeks later, at the study's conclusion, they had lost an average of 9 pounds. Far more impressive, however, were the changes in their body compositions. The average body fat percentage declined from 32.7 to 25.7 percent. This translates to 16 pounds of fat—25 percent of their initial fat mass! They also had an average reduction of 3 inches around the waist, and their fasting insulin fell by a quarter, into the normal range.[13]

These study participants were regular people who wanted to lose some weight. They were neither particularly athletic nor did they get fanatical about exercise; most of them simply walked. Their diets weren't monitored, they weren't required to count calories, and none of them reported feeling overly deprived. But the results speak for themselves. One of the men lost an astonishing 44 pounds of fat, and a 40-year-old woman lost 31 pounds of fat!

12-WEEK STUDY RESULTS (averages)

	BASELINE	WEEK 6	WEEK 12
WEIGHT (POUNDS)	198.8	192	189
BODY FAT (%)	32.7	29.8	25.7
WAIST (INCHES)	42.6	40.5	39.5
INSULIN (IU/ML)	13.2	9.0	9.9

Whitaker Wellness Study and Clinical Experience

We conducted an informal study with a similar protocol at the Whitaker Wellness Institute, recruiting overweight employees and people, male and female, from the local area. Before they began, they underwent an extensive evaluation that included weight, hip and waist measurements, a blood workup, and a body composition analysis with dual-energy x-ray absorptiometry (DXA), a sophisticated scanning device that accurately determines lean body and fat mass and bone density. The study protocol was to exercise 3 to 5 days a week, building up to 45 minutes per session, and to eat reasonably well. They received diet guidelines similar to the suggestions in Chapter 11 but weren't required to follow this or any other diet. We also provided 12 weeks' worth of the nutritional supplements you'll read about in Chapter 5. Finally, we gave them tracking forms, similar to the one in Chapter 7: Monitoring Your Progress and instructions to check in with us every week by phone or e-mail or in person.

In 12 weeks, the men, who had weighed in at an average of 220.7 pounds, lost an average of 18.3 pounds, nearly 4 inches around the waist, and almost 4 percent of their body fat, or 14.7 pounds of fat. The women's weight loss averaged 7.5 pounds, with nearly 3 inches in waist circumference and 5.4 pounds of fat. When we first crunched these numbers, we were disappointed with the outcomes among the women—until we realized that we had a few outliers whose results were so out of whack that they couldn't possibly have adhered to the program. One woman actually gained weight!

Most of the participants who followed the mini-fast with exercise program—some of whom you'll read about later in greater detail—were beyond pleased with the results. Brian lost 31 pounds in the first 8 weeks, and went on to lose 40. T.W. dropped from a size 16 to a size 12. Her clothes no longer fit, but she was reluctant to buy new ones because she planned to stay on the program and had no doubt that she would lose more. Jack lost 29 pounds and nearly 5 inches off his waist, and his wife, Stephanie, shed 13 pounds, almost all of it fat—and they both reversed their diabetes. J.G. lost a significant amount of weight and gained control of his blood sugar. And Mary, who considers herself a diet expert, since she's tried so many, declared this to be the easiest, least expensive, and most sustainable program she has ever tried.

To recap, exercising after your overnight fast and before eating, when carbohydrate stores are nearing depletion, rapidly uses

WHY THE MINI-FAST WITH EXERCISE WORKS

✔ Cuts daily caloric intake by skipping a meal

✔ Reduces the need for calorie counting and making difficult food decisions throughout the day

✔ Switches you into the fat-burning mode and keeps you there for hours

✔ Curbs appetite by triggering ketosis and eliminating blood sugar swings

✔ Allows you to eat what you want—within reason—for the rest of the day

✔ Improves underlying risk factors such as insulin resistance, inflammation, and oxidative stress, and "turns on" antiaging genes

up remaining glucose and glycogen and stimulates fat burning. Skipping breakfast and waiting until noon to eat keeps you in that mode. Until you eat again, you'll continue to burn stored fat. Provided that you don't overeat the rest of the day and that you monitor your fat intake, you will begin to chip away at your love handles and thunder thighs. This is the key to the Mini-Fast Diet: harnessing and taking advantage of the natural process of breaking down stored fat.

Don Engmann: *Winner of the* Health & Healing *Diabesity Challenge*

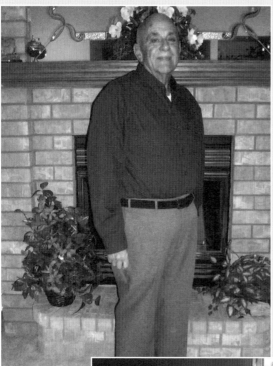

Since 1991, I've been writing *Health & Healing,* a popular monthly newsletter. After observing the success our patients at the clinic were having with the mini-fast with exercise program, I wrote about it in the newsletter. To encourage readers to give it a try, we ran a 12-week contest, which we called the Diabesity Challenge (diabetes + obesity = diabesity). The rules were simple: Skip breakfast, exercise in the morning, and take some nutritional supplements, if desired. Participants were asked to record before-and-after weights, waist and hip measurements, and, if available, blood pressure, blood sugar, cholesterol, and other markers of health.

The winner of the

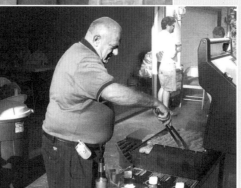

Don Engmann, before and after (above) losing 44 pounds on the mini-fast with exercise program

Diabesity Challenge was Don Engmann of Lomira, Wisconsin. His starting weight was 232 pounds. Twelve weeks later, he weighed 202, and his waist circumference had gone from 52 inches to 47. When I last spoke to Don about 6 months after the contest ended, he'd been on the mini-fast for 9 months and was still going strong. He was down to 188 pounds, for a total loss of 44 pounds, and he'd shed another 3 inches around his waist.

"I have struggled with my weight for at least 30 years," Don said, "and I've been on many diets that have not worked for me in the past. This has been the easiest program to follow. I wasn't much of an exerciser before, but now I walk for 30 to 90 minutes most every day, and I really enjoy it. I also go to the gym twice a week, and my energy level is high.

"Another nice part of the program is that you don't have to count calories— you just eat low-glycemic foods. I followed the diet to a T the first 12 weeks, but now I'll eat a small breakfast some days. My weight loss is slower at this time, but I'm continuing to lose. My goal is to get down to 175 pounds, and I'm well on my way.

"Another tremendous benefit for me has been my blood pressure. I've been on blood pressure medication for approximately 25 years, but after losing weight on the mini-fast and under my doctor's supervision, I cut back my dose over several months. As of May 10, 2011, I'm no longer on medication. My blood pressure has averaged 138/78, and I have been feeling great.

"Oh, and I've had to go shopping. When you go from a 52- to a 44-inch waist, your pants no longer fit!"

CHAPTER 4

WHY BREAKFAST *ISN'T* THE MOST IMPORTANT MEAL OF THE DAY

Here is my response to objections to skipping breakfast from people who argue that it's the most important meal of the day: "I agree. Just eat breakfast at noon!"

—JULIAN WHITAKER, MD

If cutting calories and exercising are the first and second commandments of weight loss, eating breakfast has to be the third. "Breakfast is the most important meal of the day." "Breakfast eaters are healthier." "If you skip breakfast, you'll eat more the rest of the day." "Breakfast jump-starts your metabolism." "Skipping breakfast will make you fat."

I'm here to tell you that these "truisms" just aren't true. Like a handful of other widely accepted notions in medicine, they're myths. It's not unusual for unfounded, even crazy and nonsensical ideas to become entrenched beliefs. For example, for years it was believed that tomatoes were poisonous. In 1820, a crowd gathered in New Jersey to watch a "brave and foolhardy" gentleman as he consumed one tomato after another, fully expecting him to die. He didn't, and thanks in part to this public demonstration, that particular fiction eventually faded away. But others linger. Cracking your knuckles causes arthritis. Not true. Reading in bad light ruins your eyes. Nope. We use only 10 percent of our brains. No way. Breakfast is the most important meal of the day. Absolutely false.

Nevertheless, we've heard this admonition all our lives, so we believe it. In fact, missing this deified meal is the number one initial objection to the mini-fast with exercise program. That's why I'm devoting an entire chapter in defense of skipping breakfast. As

WHO EATS BREAKFAST?

Skipping breakfast won't be much of a stretch for many people. Kellogg's, purveyor of Eggo toaster waffles, Pop-Tarts, and Frosted Flakes, recently conducted one of the largest surveys ever on the breakfast habits of Americans. After interviewing more than 14,000 people across the country, they determined that only 34 percent of us eat breakfast every day. Nearly all toddlers and preschoolers have a morning meal, as do more than three-quarters of elementary school kids. But percentages dip in middle school and high school to 50 and 35 percent, respectively. The main reason given for missing breakfast? A lack of time.[1]

you read on, you may be surprised to learn that there is little research to support this widely held conviction, especially for adults. Many highly credentialed, well-respected nutritionists and scientists agree that our infatuation with breakfast, rather than being the health-enhancing habit it's hyped up to be, is actually a significant contributor to our epidemic of obesity.

MYTH #1: SKIPPING BREAKFAST INCREASES OVERALL CALORIC INTAKE

A common contention of the pro-breakfast camp is that people who routinely skip meals make up for it by eating more throughout the day. This just doesn't make sense. Cutting out an entire meal eliminates a large chunk of calories. Even if you eat more at lunch, you're unlikely to eat a whole second meal's worth of extra food. Several studies bear this out.

In a 2011 study published in *Nutrition Journal,* German researchers tracked the food and caloric intake of 380 adults, 280 of whom were obese and 100 of normal weight. For 10 to 14 days, these people wrote down in great detail everything they ate as soon as they ate it. After tallying up daily calories, the researchers found that both heavy and slim people who ate a big breakfast had a higher total caloric intake than those who ate a small breakfast or skipped it altogether. In other words, a big breakfast did not translate into a lighter lunch or fewer snacks. It just added to the overall calorie count. The conclusion was that "overweight and obese subjects should consider the reduction of breakfast calories as a simple option to improve their daily energy balance."[2]

David Levitsky, PhD, professor of nutrition and psychology at Cornell University, came up with similar findings in an unpublished study of students at Cornell. He recruited volunteers and on some mornings served them an all-you-can-eat breakfast, while on other days they got no breakfast at all. Daily calorie consumption was recorded in both scenarios. On the no-breakfast days, the students ate approximately 150 more calories at lunch, as compared with the days they'd had a big breakfast. But food intake over the rest of the day was about the same. All told, the breakfast skippers ended up eating 450 fewer daily calories.[3]

Believe it or not, skipping breakfast actually blunts appetite for many people—and for virtually everyone if done in conjunction with exercise as part of the mini-fast, for reasons we've discussed throughout this book. However, even if you do not work out, you may find yourself less hungry in the morning on the days you don't eat. Some of this has to do with what you consume. Common morning meals include toast, bagels, pancakes, waffles, toaster pastries, and, the perennial favorite, cold cereal. High-carb, high-glycemic foods stimulate spikes in blood sugar that stimulate the release of significant amounts of insulin to clear out all that glucose. Because such foods push natural mechanisms to extremes, blood sugar may be driven too low. This phenomenon, called reactive hypoglycemia, is responsible for cravings, jitteriness, poor concentration, and other symptoms of low blood sugar that often occur between meals.

I get confirmation of this all the time from patients. Louise told me: "If I eat anything for breakfast, even a piece of whole grain toast or a bowl of cereal, I'm famished by midmorning. If I'm at home, I find myself rooting around in the fridge for more to eat, and at work I cannot resist whatever goodies are available in the break room. But when I don't eat breakfast, which is the general rule for me, and only drink coffee, I go for hours without even thinking about food."

MYTH #2: BREAKFAST EATERS HAVE SUPERIOR NUTRITIONAL STATUS

Nutritionists like to argue that breakfast is an excellent source of essential nutrients and that people who eat breakfast are better nourished. This could be true, provided that the morning meal consists of modest amounts of slow-cooked oatmeal, fresh fruit, egg whites, and other healthy foods. But that's the exception rather than the rule.

Look at the menus at IHOP, Denny's, Coco's, or any restaurant that serves breakfast. They're full of glossy, enticing pictures of eggs Benedict, stacks of pancakes with scoops of butter and syrup, three-egg cheese omelets with bacon and hash browns, French toast, cinnamon rolls, and blueberry muffins. One of these chains is now offering deep-fried funnel cakes on the breakfast menu! Granted, few of us eat like this at home, but what do we eat for breakfast? ABC News conducted a poll a few years ago and found that 2 in 10 adults eat eggs, with or without bacon; 10 percent have toast, bagels, muffins, or pastry; and a third have cold cereal. The rest eat everything from cold pizza and peanut butter sandwiches to Coke and a doughnut.[4]

But cold cereal was the clear winner. The best-selling brand in America is Cheerios—one in eight boxes of cereal sold in this country is Cheerios, which now comes in 13 different flavors, including chocolate. The most popular, and therefore the leading, breakfast food in the United States is Honey Nut Cheerios. Take a look at the box and the label of this product. The front of the box promises lower cholesterol, a reduced risk of heart disease, 13 vitamins and minerals, fiber, and whole grains. What's not to love?

Well, how about the sweeteners—9 grams (2 teaspoons) of sugar, brown sugar syrup, and honey in every ¾ cup serving? Or the measly 2 grams of fiber, which is just 7 to 8 percent of the recommended

Nutrition Facts

Serving Size ¾ cup (28g)
Servings Per Container

Amount Per Serving	Honey Nut Cheerios	with 1/2 cup skim milk
Calories	110	150
Calories from Fat	15	15

	% Daily Value**	
Total Fat 1.5g*	2%	2%
Saturated Fat 0g	0%	0%
Trans Fat 0g		
Polyunsaturated Fat 0.5g		
Monounsaturated Fat 0.5g		
Cholesterol 0mg	0%	1%
Sodium 160mg	7%	9%
Potassium 115mg	3%	9%
Total Carbohydrate 22g	7%	9%
Dietary Fiber 2g	8%	8%
Soluble Fiber less than 1g		
Sugars 9g		
Other Carbohydrate 11g		
Protein 2g		

Vitamin A	10%	15%
Vitamin C	10%	10%
Calcium	10%	25%
Iron	25%	25%
Vitamin D	10%	25%
Thiamin	25%	30%
Riboflavin	25%	35%
Niacin	25%	25%
Vitamin B$_6$	25%	25%
Folic Acid	50%	50%
Vitamin B$_{12}$	25%	35%
Phosphorus	8%	20%
Magnesium	6%	10%
Zinc	25%	30%

* Amount in cereal. A serving of cereal plus skim milk provides 1.5g total fat, less than 5 mg of cholesterol, 220mg sodium, 320mg potassium, 28g total carbohydrate (15g sugars, 12g other carbohydrate), and 7g protein.

** Percent Daily Values are based on a 2,000 calorie diet. Your daily values may be higher or lower depending on your calorie needs:

	Calories	2,000	2,500
Total Fat	Less than	65g	80g
Sat Fat	Less than	20g	25g
Cholesterol	Less than	300mg	300mg
Sodium	Less than	2,400mg	2,400mg
Potassium		3,500mg	3,500mg
Total Carbohydrate		300g	375g
Dietary Fiber		25g	30g

Ingredients: **Whole Grain Oats** (includes the oat bran), **Sugar, Modified Corn Starch, Honey, Brown Sugar Syrup, Salt, Tripotassium Phosphate, Canola and/or Rice Bran Oil, Natural Almond Flavor. Vitamin E** (mixed tocopherols) **Added to Preserve Freshness.**

Vitamins and Minerals: Calcium Carbonate, Zinc and Iron (mineral nutrients), **Vitamin C** (sodium ascorbate), **A B Vitamin** (niacinadmide), **Vitamin B$_6$** (pyridoxine hydrochloride), **Vitamin B$_2$** (riboflavin), **Vitamin B$_1$** (thiamin mononitrate), **Vitamin A** (palmitate), **A B Vitamin** (folic acid), **Vitamin B$_{12}$, Vitamin D$_3$.**

CONTAINS ALMOND; MAY CONTAIN WHEAT INGREDIENTS.

daily intake of 25 to 30 grams. Or the 2 grams of protein, which is peanuts compared with the suggested 50 to 65 grams per day. As for the 13 vitamins and minerals, they average 10 or 25 percent of the paltry RDAs. Add to this a high glycemic index and load that rapidly drive up blood sugar and lead to a crash a few hours later—and you're left feeling tired, irritable, foggy, and ravenously hungry. This is definitely not the breakfast of champions.

I'm not trying to single out Cheerios. As cold cereals go, their original cereal in the yellow box is one of the better ones on the market. And many of the other popular choices in the ABC survey—bagels, muffins, and pastries—are far worse. The point I want to make is that breakfast is not, for most people, the supernutritious meal that it's cracked up to be.

If you're trying to lose weight, you're better off skipping breakfast. You can easily make up the nutrients you may have missed by eating healthy foods the rest of the day and taking a good daily multivitamin and mineral supplement.

MYTH #3: BREAKFAST JUMP-STARTS YOUR METABOLISM

The notion that breakfast jump-starts your metabolism is just plain silly. Metabolism—the whole gamut of biochemical processes that occur within the body—doesn't need jump-starting. If it weren't always running, you'd be dead.

In terms of weight loss, metabolism is often referred to as the number of calories you burn from the breakdown of food into energy. This, too, is an ongoing process. Your basal body metabolism is the energy required to maintain normal temperature, breathe, pump blood, build and repair tissues, and accomplish the myriad other functions taking place every second to keep you alive. About 70 percent of the calories you need are expended in these crucial processes. Rates vary based on gender (men have more muscle tissue, which burns more calories), age (metabolism usually slows down as we get older and muscle mass declines), and weight (even fat requires energy to maintain).

When you eat, you do burn more calories. The process of digestion requires energy and "eats up" about 10 percent of your total daily caloric expenditure. But eating doesn't change your basal metabolic rate. You may have heard people say they can't lose weight because their metabolism is slow. It's true that some individuals do have a relatively slower or faster basal metabolic rate, but unless it's markedly affected by a medical condition—if you have hypothyroidism (low thyroid function), for example, as discussed in Chapter 8: Removing Your Roadblocks—a "sluggish metabolism" is unlikely to be the cause of your weight gain.

If you really want to jump-start your metabolism, i.e., burn more calories, skip breakfast and exercise during your mini-fast.

MYTH #4: EATING BREAKFAST IS A NATURAL, HEALTH-ENHANCING ACTIVITY

Perhaps the most vocal proponent of skipping breakfast is Mark Mattson, PhD, chief of the neurosciences lab at the National Institute on Aging. Taking the long view and looking at historical precedents, he believes that our breakfast habit is a relatively recent adaptation and is anything but natural. In an article in the *Lancet,* arguably the world's leading medical journal, he writes:

> Only until relatively recently in human evolution have we eaten three meals (plus snacks) every day. Our ancestors consumed food much less frequently, and often had to subsist on one large meal per day or go for several days at a

HOW MANY CALORIES DO YOU NEED?

A commonly used formula for determining basal metabolic rate (BMR)—how many calories you require for the basic processes that keep you alive—is called the Harris-Benedict equation. It requires a little math, so get out your calculator or go to page 144.

Men: 66 + (6.23 × weight in pounds) + (12.7 × height in inches) − (6.8 × age)
Women: 655 + (4.35 × weight in pounds) + (4.7 × height in inches) − (4.7 × age)

Here are some examples. A 30-year-old male, 5 feet 10, 180 pounds, has a BMR of 1,872, and a 6-foot, 180-pound 40-year-old man's is 1,830. A woman who is 5 feet 4, 140 pounds, and 45 years old has a BMR of 1,354. For a 25-year-old female who is 5 feet 6 and 150 pounds, it's 1,500. Note that the most significant influence on BMR is gender.

Keep your calculator handy—the Harris-Benedict equation also figures in activity level.

Sedentary (little or no exercise): BMR × 1.2
Lightly active (light exercise 1 to 3 days a week): BMR × 1.375
Moderately active (moderate exercise 3 to 5 days a week): BMR × 1.55
Very active (hard exercise 6 to 7 days a week): BMR × 1.725
Extra active (very hard exercise daily or physically active work): BMR × 1.9

This is the equation that nutritionists and dietitians often use to estimate the number of calories you require, based on your BMR and activity level, to maintain your current weight. Eating more or fewer calories should cause you to gain or lose weight. Of course, these are ballpark figures, and it is widely recognized that there is a fairly significant margin of error. However, this is the formula generally used to set calorie targets in weight loss programs.[5]

The good news about the mini-fast with exercise program is that you don't have to figure all this stuff out. You don't even have to count calories. By skipping breakfast, you will inevitably reduce your daily caloric intake, and exercising during the fasting state will turn you into a fat-burning machine.

time without food. Thus, from an evolutionary perspective, human beings were adapted to intermittent feeding rather than to grazing. Although eating three or more meals every day can promote rapid growth and sexual maturation in children, it might not be the healthiest dietary pattern for adults. Indeed, the rising tide of obesity in many developed countries occurs among individuals who consume several large meals per day. Overeating is now widely accepted as a major cause of premature death from cardiovascular disease, diabetes, and cancers, but surprisingly, few studies have determined how meal frequency affects health and disease risk. Nevertheless, individuals in the health-care professions and in the lay press have repeatedly stated that consumption of smaller and more frequent meals is healthier than that of larger and less frequent meals. This advice is given despite the lack of clear scientific evidence to justify it.

. . . Until the time that clear results are obtained in well-controlled studies, specific recommendations concerning meal frequency and health are inappropriate to make. Indeed, no clear evidence shows that the skipping of breakfast or lunch (or both) is unhealthy, and animal data suggest quite the opposite.[6]

MYTH #5: SKIPPING BREAKFAST WILL MAKE YOU FAT

To be fair, there are a number of studies that demonstrate that people who do not eat breakfast are more likely to be overweight or obese. Skeptics, however, call out both the quality of these studies and their lack of definitive conclusions. You also have to keep in mind that many of the breakfast studies have been funded by cereal manufacturers, the American Egg Board, and the like, and it is generally recognized that industry-sponsored research tends to shine a flattering light on industry products. I'm not saying they're out to scam us, but this tendency, called experimenter bias, holds true in all fields of research.

As Dr. Mattson points out in the *Lancet* article, the bulk of the research shows no clear association between skipping breakfast or other meals and weight gain or any other adverse health outcome. Common sense, backed by animal studies and a small but growing body of human research, suggests that the opposite is true.

I am not recommending that you send your kids off to school with nothing to eat. A child's attention, performance, and overall nutritional status may well benefit from having breakfast. But for adults and perhaps older children who are trying to lose weight, skipping the morning meal is a relatively easy way to reduce overall caloric intake.

BREAKFAST IS THE EASIEST MEAL TO MISS

As you've learned, skipping breakfast is a central component of the mini-fast with exercise. The whole point of the program—of any

NEVER ATE BREAKFAST, NEVER BEEN OVERWEIGHT

Here's an e-mail I recently received from K.M. of Silver Peak, Nevada: "Unknowingly, I have been practicing the 'mini-fast' most of my life. I have never wanted to eat until noon. My parents and friends have nagged me throughout the years, saying, 'You have to eat breakfast. It's the most important meal of the day!' I ignored them all, and have *never* been overweight in my 64 years of life despite my healthy appetite. Keep up the good work, Doc!"

weight loss program worth its salt—is to burn stored fat, and as I've said repeatedly throughout this book, there are only three ways to accomplish this:

1. Significantly reduce calories

2. Dramatically increase exercise

3. Exercise moderately in the fasting state when no carbohydrates are available for energy, insulin levels are at their lowest, and the body naturally switches to burning fat, i.e., mini-fast with exercise

Of course, you could eat breakfast and a light lunch, fast in the afternoon and evening, and exercise late in the day. Or you could have an early breakfast, skip lunch, exercise in the afternoon, then eat a light dinner. (These are all options that will be discussed in the next chapter.) The point is to exercise when your glucose and glycogen stores are near exhaustion so that your body will turn to burning fat for energy. This only happens hours after your last meal—and ends when you eat again.

The reason I emphasize forgoing breakfast and exercising in the morning is because most people find that it's easier that way. You've already been fasting for 10 to 12 hours while you were asleep, and you did it without even trying. Avoiding food for long stretches during the day requires discipline; nighttime fasting does not. Breakfast is also the most convenient meal to skip. Dinner, for most of us, is a time to relax, unwind, and enjoy the company of our family and friends. Lunch, depending on your individual circumstances, may not be much of a social event. However, if you are at work or otherwise out and about, you are likely to be surrounded by the smells of food, the sight of people dining, and other temptations to eat. Breakfast tends to be the most solitary meal of the day, the one we eat on the run and, in terms of relaxation or socialization, enjoy the least. If breakfast foods are your favorite, I can relate—there's nothing better than an omelet or a couple of eggs with a little turkey bacon. So do what I do: eat "breakfast" for lunch or dinner.

Mark McCarty, the researcher who came up with the original concept of the mini-fast with exercise program, summed it up beautifully in a recent conversation.

I have always preferred the morning version of mini-fast with exercise—the one that the Whitaker Wellness Institute is now recommending—because your evening of sleep is an *effortless enforced fast.* When you wake up, your free fatty acid levels are as high as they will be all day, ripe for burning! Plus, when I wake up I feel energized and ready for exercise, whereas when I get home after a day's work, my

COFFEE IS MORE THAN OKAY

When I told a good friend about the mini-fast with exercise program, his first question was, "Can I have my morning coffee?" It was the one condition that had to be met before he would even consider giving it a shot. My answer was an enthusiastic *yes!*

It is perfectly acceptable to drink coffee, tea, water, or any noncaloric beverage during the fasting hours of this program. In fact, there are advantages to getting some caffeine in your system prior to working out. It helps mobilize stored fat and facilitates fat burning, even in the presence of glycogen. This glycogen-sparing effect enhances endurance exercise, which is the kind of activity you'll be doing as a part of this program.

Adding a lot of sugar and milk would obviously defeat the purpose of morning fasting. Some of the specialty drinks at Starbucks and other coffee shops contain upwards of 300 calories and 30 to 40 grams of carbohydrates, most of it from sugar. On the other hand, flavoring your coffee or tea with a calorie-free sweetener and a little creamer isn't going to break the bank. So enjoy your morning pick-me-up in good conscience. By the way, my friend, the coffee fiend, started the program and within 4 months lost about 15 pounds.

urge is to drink a good beer and veg out in front of the TV. But if there are reasons morning exercise isn't practical for you, other variants may be a good alternative.

WHAT, HOW MUCH—NOT WHEN

I want to end with a quote from Marion Nestle, PhD, professor in the department of nutrition, food studies, and public health at New York University and one of the country's best-known nutritionists. In her book *What to Eat,* Dr. Nestle maintains: "I am well aware that everyone says breakfast is the most important meal of the day, but I am not convinced. What you eat—and how much—matters more to your health than when you eat."[7]

And remember, I'm not saying that breakfast is unimportant— just eat it at noon!

Roxie Tanner: "I Am Now at My Ideal Weight, and I Plan to Stay There"

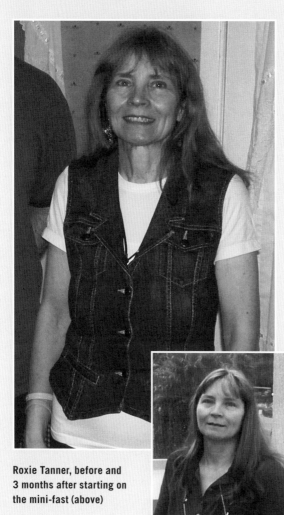

Roxie Tanner, before and 3 months after starting on the mini-fast (above)

"I have been healthy most of my life. The only things of significance in my medical history were the births of my two sons and a noncancerous lump in my thyroid. I do take medication for my thyroid, and although my thyroid hormone levels fluctuate, it is under reasonably good control.

"Throughout my childhood and early adult life, my weight was normal. In my late twenties, I started gaining weight due to bad food choices, lack of exercise, and stress. I tried many diets, which would work for a short time, and then I would gain the weight back. In 2004, I went to my doctor for a minor matter, and when they weighed me, I was 196 pounds! My blood pressure was also high.

"When I came home from that appointment, I decided that it was time to make some changes in my eating habits and lifestyle. I became a vegan on June 23, 2004—a day that is as important to me as my birthday. I began eating mostly raw veggies and fruits, plus pasta, bread, legumes, and soy products. It's been pretty easy because there are so many vegan options out there now, although some of them are high in calories and fat. I also started walking once or twice a day and used an exercise bike when I couldn't walk outside. On the vegan diet, I eventually got my weight down to 143 pounds, which was a lot to lose but still too much for my height of 5 feet 3.

"I read about the mini-fast with exercise in Dr. Whitaker's newsletter, which I have received for years, and started it on January 9, 2010. By April 20, I had lost 20 pounds! I am very pleased with this program. It really is not that hard to do. The first day I just pretended I was fasting for my blood work. Now, going without breakfast feels normal to me. When I go on vacation, I usually eat when everyone else is eating, but I get right back on the program as soon as I get home.

"For anyone thinking about doing this, I want to say that I consider the mini-fast with exercise program to be a life plan rather than a diet. You still have to eat reasonably and exercise, which you should be doing anyway, but with this program it pays off. This has been the easiest way for me to lose weight and keep it off. I have read about others who lost 30 or more pounds, so this program is good for those who need to lose a large amount of weight. Had I known about it in 2004 when I became a vegan, I am sure I would have been able to get the weight off much faster. But it is also very effective for those like me who were looking to lose less. I am now at my ideal weight, and I plan to stay there."

PART II

The Mini-Fast with Exercise Program

I've tried your mini-fast program for almost 7 months now, with terrific results! I've reduced my weight from 210 to 196, mostly around the middle, and agree that it has been easily implemented, simple, logical, and inexpensive. I have always had a regular physical activity routine and eaten a well-balanced diet, so the only difference was eliminating breakfast.

—HARRY WILLWATER

CHAPTER 5

GETTING STARTED

If you do not change direction, you may end up where you are heading.

—LAO TZU, CHINESE PHILOSOPHER,
6TH CENTURY BCE

The groundwork for the mini-fast with exercise has been established. You now know what makes this program unique and how it fills the gaps and sidesteps the hazards of most weight loss approaches. You understand why it works from a scientific perspective, that it taps into and accelerates the body's natural fat-burning mechanisms. You have a better appreciation for the reasons behind our epidemic of obesity and why slimming down is so difficult yet so rewarding. You've read and will continue to read how people like you finally found in the mini-fast with exercise not a short-term diet but a true solution to their weight problems and a healthy lifestyle that they can stick with indefinitely.

As I've said before, this program does not require you to go out and spend a lot of money. There are no special foods or exercise equipment to buy, and although the nutritional supplements we'll discuss later in this chapter are helpful, they are 100 percent optional. Just skip a meal, exercise while mini-fasting, and eat sensibly the rest of the day—that's it.

Right now, today, at this very moment, you have everything you need to embark on the mini-fast with exercise and begin to reap the program's tremendous benefits. All that's left is for you to make a decision, commit to it, and get started.

WHEN AND HOW TO EXERCISE

Here are a few key points to keep in mind in order to get optimal results with the mini-fast with exercise program.

Select an exercise activity or activities. Because the goal is to get rid of stored fat, you need to choose an aerobic activity, which, by definition, is exercise of moderate intensity and relatively long duration. Prolonged moderate-intensity exercise suppresses insulin, mobilizes fat, and sets the stage for fat burning—fat burning that will persist for several hours after exercise, provided that you continue to fast. Examples include brisk walking, jogging, wogging (a combination of walking and jogging), stair climbing, cycling, swimming, using an elliptical glider or a stair-stepper, taking an aerobics class, and playing singles tennis or other racquet sports. Weight-bearing exercise is preferable, but if you have bad knees, riding a stationary bike, cycling, or swimming is fine. Walking is by far the most popular activity because practically anyone can do it, and all it requires is putting on your shoes and heading out the door. To avoid boredom, which often leads to giving up exercise altogether, I suggest mixing up your activities. Strength training is also desirable, as it builds muscle, and the more muscle you have, the higher your basal metabolic rate and the more calories you burn at rest. But focus on aerobic activities or interval routines that involve both aerobic and strengthening exercises during your mini-fast.

Exercise while you are fasting. Morning exercisers skip breakfast and eat nothing until around lunchtime. Midday exercisers omit lunch and snacks between breakfast and dinner. The evening option involves eating breakfast, lunch, and perhaps an afternoon snack but omitting both dinner and snacking before bedtime. Should none of these options be acceptable and you are unwilling to forgo a meal, then build a window of fasting around your exercise: a minimum of 2 hours without food before exercise and as many hours as possible afterward. But remember, the longer the fasting period, the more efficiently you will burn fat.

Work out at moderate intensity. Moderate aerobic activity—not too slow and not too intense—for a protracted period is ideal for burning fat. Your heart rate and cardiovascular demands should increase, and you should work up a sweat, but you should also be able to carry on a normal conversation while exercising. (The target intensity level is 60 to 80 percent of your maximum heart rate, which I'll tell you more about in Chapter 10.)[1] If you are deconditioned, it won't take much at first to get you huffing and puffing, so go easy and build up gradually. A leisurely walk around the block may be all you can handle right now; so be it. As you keep it up and become better trained, you will naturally increase your intensity.

Aim for at least 40 minutes of exercise. To maximize fat burning, try to exercise for a minimum of 40 minutes per session. Of course, you will need to ease into this—the last thing you want to do is sustain an injury or burn yourself out before you really get started. If you have been inactive, 5 minutes may be your initial goal. But as your muscle tone and cardiovascular fitness improve, steadily increase the duration of your sessions to 40 minutes or more. There will be days when your schedule is such that you can squeeze in only 20 or 30 minutes. Just do your best and know that anything is better than nothing.

Exercise three to five times a week. I suggest that you set a goal of 5 days of exercise a week. I understand you won't always be able to fit in every session, and if you miss a day, don't beat yourself up. However, it's better to aim high than to go for the bare minimum. Once you get down to your ideal weight, you may be able to ease up on your exercise frequency, but strive to engage in some type of activity no fewer than 3 days per week, regardless of your weight.

Drink plenty of water and perhaps some coffee or tea before and after exercise. Staying hydrated is obviously important, and on the days you exercise, you'll require extra fluids. Water is your best choice. A cup of coffee or tea before exercise, with or without low-calorie creamer and calorie-free sweetener, is also recommended. Caffeine enhances fat mobilization and utilization and helps sustain aerobic endurance.[2] Although these effects aren't overly significant, they work in synergy with the mini-fast with exercise.

WHEN AND WHAT TO EAT

When I said that this is actually not a diet, I meant it. Stick to these tips and you'll have no problem eating well and losing weight.

Eat whenever you want—except during your mini-fast. For most of you, this means abstaining from eating until noon. If you elect to exercise at a time of day other than in the morning, avoid eating for several hours before and after you exercise—the longer the fasting period, the more efficient and prolonged the fat burning. For instance, if you exercise at noon, eat breakfast and a late dinner, or if you exercise in the late afternoon or evening, have

(continued on page 94)

HOW TO SCHEDULE YOUR MINI-FAST

As I've said before, skipping breakfast as part of the mini-fast with exercise is the easiest because you've already been fasting while you slept. For many people, exercising in the morning before the hectic day begins is also more convenient.

But this program will work with any schedule, so if mornings aren't good for you, it's still a fantastic way to lose weight. Just be aware that this will require skipping lunch or dinner in order to exercise while fasting. If you simply cannot miss a meal, then select a time to exercise that is as long as possible (at least 2 hours) after eating, when your insulin level is low, and do not eat for as long as possible afterward.

Also, don't feel locked into a particular schedule. You are by no means required to exercise at the same time every day. You may elect to exercise in the mornings during the week, for instance, but at noon on weekends. This is your program; make it work with your schedule.

To give you an idea of how these various scheduling options might work out, here are some scenarios of typical days on the mini-fast.

You'll notice references to Ketosis Essentials and Metabolic Essentials. Ketosis Essentials is a powder mixed in water and taken before exercise to boost exercise endurance and facilitate fat burning. You can take it again during your fasting period to help curb your appetite. Metabolic Essentials is a supplement taken with meals to enhance weight loss and improve multiple aspects of metabolic syndrome. Taking these weight loss aids is optional; you could take one but not the other, you could take one just occasionally, you could take other supplements with similar ingredients, or you could take nothing at all. I describe them in more detail starting on page 97.

Morning Exercise

6:00 a.m.   Wake up.

6:15 a.m.   Drink a cup of coffee, tea, or water.

6:30 a.m.   Wog (walk/jog) for 45 minutes. If desired, take Ketosis Essentials.

7:15 a.m.   Shower, dress, go to work.

10:00 a.m.   Have coffee, tea, or other calorie-free beverage but no food. If desired, take another dose of Ketosis Essentials.

12:00 p.m.   Eat lunch. If desired, take Metabolic Essentials.

3:30 p.m.   Have a snack and/or beverage of your choice.

7:30 p.m.   Eat dinner. If desired, take another dose of Metabolic Essentials.

10:30 p.m.   Go to bed.

Afternoon Exercise

7:00 a.m.   Wake up.

7:15 a.m.   Eat breakfast. If desired, take Metabolic Essentials.

7:45 a.m.   Shower, dress, go to work.

10:00 a.m.   Have coffee, tea, or other calorie-free beverage but no food.

12:00 p.m.   Walk briskly for 45 minutes. If desired, take Ketosis Essentials.

3:30 p.m.   Have coffee, tea, or another calorie-free beverage but no food. If desired, take another dose of Ketosis Essentials.

6:30 p.m.   Eat dinner. If desired, take another dose of Metabolic Essentials.

11:00 p.m.   Go to bed.

Evening Exercise

8:00 a.m.   Wake up.

8:30 a.m.   Have breakfast. If desired, take Metabolic Essentials.

9:00 a.m.   Shower, dress, go to work.

10:30 a.m.   Have a snack and/or beverage of your choice.

12:30 p.m.   Eat lunch. If desired, take another dose of Metabolic Essentials.

3:30 p.m.   Have a snack and/or beverage of your choice.

6:00 p.m.   Go to the gym and walk on the treadmill or take an aerobics class for 45 minutes. If desired, take Ketosis Essentials.

7:30 p.m.   Have decaf tea or another calorie-free beverage but no food. If desired, take another dose of Ketosis Essentials.

11:30 p.m.   Go to bed.

breakfast and lunch. (See pages 92–93 for sample schedules.) Although it isn't as important to fast on days when you don't exercise, most people who have succeeded on this program find that skipping a meal every day reinforces the habit and is an easy way to reduce calories.

Drink water and other calorie-free beverages during the fasting period and throughout the day. It's always important to drink a lot of water, and if you are a coffee or tea drinker, I highly recommend it before exercising, as discussed above, as well as during morning and perhaps early afternoon fasting periods. (Caffeine in the late afternoon and evening may interfere with sleep.) Low-calorie creamer and calorie-free sweeteners are acceptable, but don't add honey, sugar, or other sweeteners—and strictly avoid lattes, mochas, and other milky, flavored coffee drinks. They can contain as many calories and carbohydrates as a small meal! In addition to its positive effects on exercise and fat burning, caffeine also curbs appetite to a mild degree. Furthermore, sipping coffee, tea, or another beverage gives you something to do with your hands and put in your mouth. Much of the "hunger" we experience is really just the habit and enjoyment of eating. Drinking your favorite beverages while mini-fasting is a treat that is not only allowed but encouraged. I cannot in good conscience advocate diet sodas and artificial sweeteners, but in reality any calorie-free beverage will do.

Eat sensibly the rest of the day. Don't feel like you have to count calories—this program is really about turning on your fat-burning furnace by exercising during a window of fasting. But you do need to use common sense and some degree of self-restraint when it comes to food. You can't expect to trim down by skipping one meal, then making up for it at the next one. Gluttony will undermine any program. The mini-fast with exercise is not a diet in the usual sense of the word, so there's nothing you have to eat and nothing that is strictly off-limits. However, if you've been eating a standard American diet (low in vegetables, fiber, and whole foods and high in saturated fat, fried, and processed items, sugars, and refined grains), this is a good time to make some changes. The people who get the best and quickest results are generally those who are compliant with mini-fasting and exercise but also eat reasonably well.

Avoid excess dietary fat. Much of the fat that ends up on our bellies and rear ends comes from the fat we eat, so it's best to limit your intake of calorie-dense dietary fats. Saturated fat, found primarily in meat and other animal-derived foods, has a negative impact on insulin sensitivity, which is a perennial problem for most overweight individuals. When saturated fat impairs the muscle cells' ability to respond to insulin, your pancreas compensates by secreting more and more insulin. Insulin is the hormone that signals your fat cells to take up, store, and retain fat. It's no accident that people who habitually consume a diet with a low ratio of saturated to unsaturated fat—Mediterranean or vegan diets, for example—tend to be relatively lean, even if their diets aren't low in fat overall. No one expects you to become a vegetarian or a vegan, but do limit your saturated fat intake by eating lean meat, skinless poultry, reduced-fat dairy products, and mostly egg whites (one whole egg per day, up to seven a week, is fine). The healthiest dietary fats are monounsaturated (olive oil, avocados, almonds, and hazelnuts) and omega-3s (salmon and other fish). Paying attention to your fat intake while on the mini-fast with exercise program will make weight loss a cinch.

Include protein with every meal and snack. Protein minimizes insulin secretion and helps control appetite, which is why I suggest that you include protein-rich items with all meals and snacks. This doesn't mean you have to follow a very high-protein diet. Serving sizes of 20 to 30 grams (4 to 6 ounces) with meals, and half that for snacks, are adequate. To limit saturated fat intake, go for lean protein sources such as fish, egg whites, low-fat dairy, skinless chicken and turkey, beans, and legumes.

Eat lots of plant foods. Fiber-rich vegetables, beans, and legumes should be dietary mainstays. Low in calories and loaded with nutrients, they fill you up, not out. You simply cannot have too many vegetables—it's virtually impossible to get fat on spinach and zucchini. Fruit is higher in sugar than veggies are, so eat it more moderately, a couple of pieces a day for most people and even less if you have diabetes (depending on your blood sugar response). I also recommend avoiding fruit juice for the most part,

THE MINI-FAST WITH EXERCISE PROGRAM AT-A-GLANCE GUIDE

✔ Select an exercise activity (or activities).

✔ Exercise while you are fasting.

✔ Work out at moderate intensity.

✔ Aim for at least 40 minutes of exercise per session.

✔ Exercise three to five times a week.

✔ Drink plenty of water and coffee or tea, if desired, before exercising.

✔ Eat whenever you want—except during your mini-fast.

✔ Continue to drink water and other calorie-free beverages during the fasting period and throughout the day.

✔ Eat sensibly the rest of the day.

✔ Limit your intake of fatty foods, especially those high in saturated fat.

✔ Include protein with every meal and snack.

✔ Eat lots of plant foods.

✔ Go easy on processed foods.

✔ Drink alcohol moderately, if at all.

as it is a highly concentrated source of sugar and calories. As for grains, make sure that they're whole and have them in moderation.

Go easy on high-glycemic refined carbohydrates and processed foods. Refined grains, sugars, and the processed foods made with them such as breads, cold cereals, crackers, cookies, chips, and sodas can sabotage the most earnest weight loss efforts. These nutrient-depleted foods have a high glycemic index, so they cause blood sugar peaks and valleys that stimulate food cravings and keep insulin levels elevated. Refined carbs plus added fats are the primary ingredients in thousands of processed foods such as desserts, frozen dinners, snacks, and restaurant fare that are convenient, inexpensive, tasty, and incredibly easy to overindulge in. If there's one diet change you make, let it be cutting back on processed foods.

Drink alcohol moderately, if at all. If you enjoy wine, beer, or other alcoholic beverages, go ahead and have, at most, a drink or two a day. The health benefits of modest amounts of alcohol are well established. In fact, studies show that women who drink regularly and responsibly are less likely to gain weight than teetotalers.[3] Be aware that alcohol puts the brakes on fat burning, so it should never be consumed during your fasting period. And alcohol abuse is devastating on many, many levels, so know your limits.

SUPPLEMENTS THAT PROMOTE FAT BURNING AND EASE FASTING

The real power of the mini-fast with exercise is its ability to jump-start fat burning, which is the only path to meaningful weight loss. Mark McCarty, the researcher who originated this concept and has been refining it for 15 years, has experimented with dozens of diet strategies, exercise regimens, and other elements to enhance the program's benefits and make it easier to follow. Years ago, Mark came up with a nutritional supplement program that is the perfect adjunct to the mini-fast with exercise: It boosts energy and fat metabolism *and* reduces the hunger pangs and discomfort that may be experienced during fasting.[4]

I've personally used the supplement that Mark formulated, and I found that it truly did make a difference, especially in terms of appetite. When I took it before exercise, no matter what time of day, I simply was not hungry. The downside? It was bulky, so it required either a lot of capsules—more than most people are willing to take—or a powder that didn't taste all that great. It was also hard on sensitive gastrointestinal tracts.

Ketosis Essentials

Mark and I combined our efforts and came up with something that is even more effective than the original formula, plus it tastes better and is better tolerated. We call it Ketosis Essentials, and it contains four main ingredients that work together to turn your fat-burning furnace up and your appetite down.

Hydroxycitric acid (HCA) is an herbal extract from the rind of a fruit called *Garcinia cambogia,* which has a long history of traditional use in India. HCA is ideal for the mini-fast with exercise program because it stimulates the activity of an enzyme that enables fat to be burned in the liver. It also boosts the production of ketones, which fuel the brain and reduce the food cravings, irritability, fatigue, and concentration difficulties that can occur with fasting. To top it off, HCA improves exercise endurance.[5]

Several clinical studies have demonstrated HCA's benefits. In a placebo-controlled study, researchers at Georgetown University Medical School put overweight men and women on a 2,000-calorie diet and had them do 30 minutes of exercise 5 days a week. They were also randomly placed in one of three supplement groups: The first group received 2,800 milligrams of HCA; those in the second group took 2,800 milligrams of HCA, along with chromium and *Gymnema sylvestre*; and those in the third group were given placebos. When they were reevaluated after 8 weeks, insignificant changes were noted in the placebo group. Both HCA groups, however, reported reductions in appetite and lost 5 to 6 percent of their total body weight. They also had improvements in cholesterol, triglyceride, and leptin levels.[6]

When HCA came on the market a few years ago, it was heralded as the best appetite suppressant and weight loss supplement ever. But it eventually lost its luster, and I can tell you why. Most of the studies used daily doses of 1,000 to 2,800 milligrams.[7] Yet typical supplements on the market contain 250 milligrams of HCA, with instructions to take it two or three times a day. A dose of Ketosis Essentials contains 1,800 milligrams of HCA, and it may be taken once or twice a day.

L-carnitine, another ingredient in Ketosis Essentials, amplifies HCA's effects. Carnitine is a naturally occurring amino acid involved in fat metabolism. The bulk of the fat stored in our adipose tissue is long-chain fatty acids. In order for them to get into the mitochondria, where energy is produced, they must first be attached to carnitine. An enzyme called carnitine palmitoyl transferase-1 (CPT-1) is required before carnitine and fatty acids can hook up.[8]

When you're eating normally, you have robust insulin levels and glycogen reserves and your body is primed to use glucose for energy. Therefore, carnitine stores and CPT-1 activity in the liver are limited. However, when you fast, carnitine migrates from the muscles to the liver and CPT-1 activity steps up to transport more fatty acids into the mitochondria, where they are rapidly burned for energy. This adaptation usually takes a few days, which explains why the first couple of days on a total fast are difficult, but on about day 3, hunger eases and energy picks up. Taking supplemental L-carnitine simply increases carnitine stores in the liver, which shortcuts and speeds up this usually slow transition to fat burning. That is carnitine's contribution to making the mini-fast with exercise easier to tolerate and fat metabolism more efficient. Each dose of Ketosis Essentials, which is to be taken once or twice daily, contains 500 milligrams.

Chromium is a trace mineral that enhances the activity of insulin and is involved in carbohydrate, fat, and protein metabolism. It also has ameliorating effects on blood sugar and is therefore particularly beneficial for those with type 2 diabetes or metabolic syndrome, which includes most people with abdominal obesity. Research also shows that one form of chromium, chromium picolinate, reduces hunger and food cravings.[9] Taken alone, chromium has a modest but observable effect on weight loss,[10] but it's a key part of the overall strategy. Ketosis Essentials contains 200 micrograms of chromium picolinate per dose.

Glycine is a sweet-tasting amino acid that triggers the release of glucagon, a hormone that turns on fat burning in the liver and generates pyruvate, a natural compound required for the production of ATP. Supplemental pyruvate in very large doses has been shown to facilitate weight loss, but in these hefty amounts it's quite pricey and can cause gastrointestinal side effects. Because glycine is converted into pyruvate, it is an inexpensive, well-tolerated stand-in. This amino acid boasts other benefits as well, including reducing inflammation and protecting against diabetic complications of the eyes, kidneys, and other organs. Approximately 4,000 milligrams per dose is required to adequately boost pyruvate levels and affect fat metabolism.

The glycine research is very new. However, HCA, carnitine, chromium, and pyruvate have been shown to be extremely effective in initiating fat loss. In a 30-day clinical trial, obese participants were required to exercise in a fasting state and eat a reasonable diet—in other words, follow the mini-fast with exercise program—and take supplements containing 1,500 milligrams of HCA, 250 milligrams of L-carnitine, 600 milligrams of chromium picolinate, and 12 grams of calcium pyruvate. In just 4 weeks, they lost an average of 13.2 pounds. More remarkable, their lean-tissue-to-fat ratio dramatically improved. All told, they shed an average of 5 pounds of fat and added 1.76 pounds of lean muscle mass per week![11]

To recap, the HCA-carnitine-chromium-glycine combo is a perfect partner for the mini-fast with exercise program. It accelerates fat burning, blunts appetite, makes fasting more tolerable, and improves exercise endurance—exactly what we're trying to accomplish. Each dose of Ketosis Essentials contains 1,800 milligrams of HCA, 500 milligrams of L-carnitine, 200 micrograms of chromium, and 4,000 milligrams of glycine. For mini-fasters and exercisers, I recommend mixing one scoop in water prior to working out during the mini-fasting period. If hunger is an issue after exercise and before your first meal several hours later, a second dose may be taken.

Metabolic Essentials

Because so many of my patients who are overweight are also afflicted with metabolic syndrome, which we discussed in Chapter 2, I formulated another supplement to address several aspects of this very common cluster of conditions: abdominal obesity, lipid abnormalities, high blood pressure, and insulin resistance. If you are struggling with any of these, consider adding Metabolic

LOST 17 POUNDS, METABOLIC SYNDROME UNDER CONTROL

H.N., from Atlanta, is a *Health & Healing* subscriber who wrote: "I have had metabolic syndrome for at least 20 years. I started on your mini-fast with exercise (only a cup of coffee instead of breakfast, and no food until lunch). My initial weight was 265. Now, less than 3 months later, it's 248—a drop of 17 pounds—and I am keeping it off without a struggle, just with a commitment to follow this simple regimen. My appetite is reduced; I rarely even want anything before lunch, and I eat less for lunch and dinner as well. I have no doubt I will reach my weight loss goal within several months. Thank you for showing me the way to manage my metabolic syndrome."

Essentials, a supplement that's meant to be taken twice a day with meals.

GreenSelect, an extract of decaffeinated green tea (*Camellia sinensis*) rich in catechins and particularly epigallocatechin gallate (EGCG), is the star ingredient in Metabolic Essentials. EGCG and other catechins are potent antioxidants and have numerous health benefits, particularly for the cardiovascular and immune systems. Studies also suggest that they have advantages for anyone trying to lose weight, including increasing fat burning, reducing appetite, and upregulating enzymes involved in fatty acid oxidation in the liver.[12] The catechins in GreenSelect are particularly impressive because they are bound to phosphatidylcholine, which dramatically increases absorption.

In a placebo-controlled study, Italian researchers recruited 100 obese men and women, ages 25 to 60, and placed them on reduced-calorie diets: 1,850 calories per day for men, and 1,350 for women. For 90 days, all of the study participants followed these dietary guidelines, but half of them also took 300 milligrams per day of GreenSelect (the amount in Metabolic Essentials), while the other half took placebo capsules. The results were astonishing. In 3 months, the men taking the green tea extract lost an average of 34 pounds, and the women an average of 26 pounds. Significant improvements were also noted in their cholesterol, triglycerides, leptin, and cortisol levels. Those in the placebo group who were simply on a low-cal diet lost an average of 10 pounds.[13]

Metabolic Essentials also contains 500 milligrams of Amla (*Emblica officinalis*), a classic remedy in Ayurveda, the traditional medicine system of India. Amla has been demonstrated in clinical trials to improve blood sugar control, increase protective HDL cholesterol, and lower LDL cholesterol, triglycerides, and C-reactive protein (CRP), a marker of inflammation and an independent risk factor for heart disease.[14]

To further lower insulin resistance and improve blood sugar control, I added 1,000 milligrams of an extract of another Ayurvedic herb, ivy gourd (*Coccinia cordifolia*). In a 90-day, double-blind, placebo-controlled clinical trial, 60 people who had been recently diagnosed with type 2 diabetes took either 1,000 milligrams of coccinia extract or a placebo. Those who took this herb had a 15.6 percent decrease in fasting blood glucose and significant declines in hemoglobin A1C, an indicator of longer-term blood sugar control.[15]

Metabolic Essentials also contains 250 milligrams of magnesium and 400 IU of vitamin D_3. Magnesium relaxes the arteries and plays a central role in blood pressure regulation and cardiovascular health.[16] Vitamin D deficiencies—which run rampant in this country—are implicated in a wide range of health challenges, including obesity, insulin resistance, metabolic syndrome, and type 2 diabetes.[17]

Helpful but Not Necessary

Let me make it clear that taking these or other supplements is completely optional.* Many people who adhere to the Mini-Fast Diet think these supplements are indispensable; some took them for a time but didn't feel they made much of a difference and discontinued them; and others never tried them at all. We offered them to participants in our study and had the same feedback—good, bad, and indifferent. Yet all these individuals have had and are continuing to have excellent success with the program.

I suggest that you go ahead and get started on the regimen, and if you find hunger or other adverse symptoms of fasting getting the best of you, then give the supplements a try. You'll find additional suggestions for overcoming appetite in the next chapter, Staying on Track.

THE MINI-FAST IN REAL LIFE

Now let's see how the mini-fast with exercise plays out in real life. I'm going to walk you through a day in the life of a typical mini-faster. Hal, as I'll call him, is the husband of one of my co-workers. He is extremely enthusiastic about this program, but he's also a very private person who doesn't want to share his pictures or use his real name. But in every other respect, his story is factual.

Hal gets up in the morning around 5:30, puts on his sweats, and sits down at his computer to check e-mails. He drinks a cup of coffee and skims the newspaper, then laces up his running shoes and heads out to exercise. Some mornings he jogs on a bike trail near his house; other days he walks on the beach with his wife. He recently added a jump-rope, pushup, and situp routine to mix it up a bit. These morning exercise sessions last 30 minutes to

*Ketosis Essentials and Metabolic Essentials are available from Whitaker Wellness (800–810–6655, www.whitakerwellness.com). It is not my intention to make a hard sell for these particular products. If you can find other supplements with similar ingredients, feel free to substitute.

an hour, and he averages 4 to 5 days a week. Then he showers, gets dressed, and settles into his home office to work.

During the morning, he wanders into the kitchen for a couple of more cups of coffee, but he doesn't eat or feel hungry. At noon, he breaks his fast for the first time, usually with leftovers, a sandwich, a can of soup, or sometimes a homemade smoothie. He goes out about once a week to meet clients for lunch, and when he does, he orders whatever sounds good, generally something with chicken or fish, since he's not much of a meat eater.

In the early afternoon, he drinks more coffee and may have a midafternoon snack, perhaps a piece of fruit, a granola bar, or a couple of cookies. Around 6:00, he knocks off work and has a glass of wine or a beer and a handful of nuts or pretzels as he chats with his wife while she prepares dinner. They are on no special diet, but she is health-conscious and cooks accordingly. Hal has learned to watch his portion sizes and usually passes on second helpings, but he has a ferocious sweet tooth—and he indulges it. Within 3 months of starting the program, he lost 15 pounds and got down to his target weight. Eight months later, he's still there and has had no trouble maintaining either his weight or the program.

Hal is a typical mini-faster. He isn't perfect—cookies, desserts, and pretzels aren't on anyone's top 10 list of healthy foods. But like many people who have success on the mini-fast, he has made it work for him. "My Achilles' heel," he says, "is my sweet tooth. My grandmother lived with us when I was growing up, and she was always baking something. To me, a meal isn't really complete without some kind of dessert. That's one reason why I like this program. If I had been told I could never eat sweets, there's no way I would have given this the time of day. But cutting out breakfast, exercising 4 or 5 days a week, and eating less at mealtime allow me to eat dessert and not regain the weight."

Hal's dessert trade-off is just one example of how people have successfully personalized the program to accommodate what matters to them. A wide range of diet strategies have been adopted. Michael is a self-avowed meat eater who, like Hal and his desserts, wouldn't have stuck with a diet that didn't allow hamburgers and steaks. Roxie, on the other hand, is a vegan; and others have found that a low-carb approach suits them best. Steve has adapted to eating most meals out, and John's solution was to order meals prepared by a chef and delivered to his home.

Exercise routines vary as well. Early-morning Jazzercize classes, midmorning walks pushing kids in a stroller, sessions with a personal trainer, lunchtime jaunts around the block with fellow workers: All are examples of successful exercise strategies that have been adopted by mini-fasters. Timing can also be tailored for individual preferences and needs. Louise has no problem doing without breakfast, but by 10:30 or 11:00, she's hungry. Even though she doesn't hold out until noon, she maintains her normal weight. Conversely, I sometimes eliminate both breakfast and lunch and eat only dinner, especially when I take a second dose of the supplements. I just forget to eat!

The point I want to make is that the "rules" are not set in stone. The mini-fast with exercise can be customized for most all lifestyles, food and activity preferences, schedules, and health and fitness levels. Don't believe me? Then read on for answers to the most common objections we hear from patients and others contemplating the program.

OVERCOMING OBJECTIONS

There is no end to the number of roadblocks you could throw out as excuses for not trying the mini-fast with exercise—or even considering it. Believe me, I've heard them all. Although I attempt to address them throughout the book, I want to respond to the most common objections here and now.

"**I can't go without breakfast.**" Not to be flippant, but have you ever tried? And if you have, I doubt if you've done it in the context of the Mini-Fast Diet. You'll be surprised at how effectively fat burning—which is what happens when you skip breakfast and exercise in the morning—holds off hunger and maintains energy.

Nevertheless, the idea that skipping breakfast is somehow harmful or unhealthy is such a widespread belief that I've written an entire chapter dispelling the popular but unfounded myth that breakfast is the most important meal of the day. Truth is, forgoing breakfast does not lead to overeating, poor nutrition, or weight gain. In fact, studies suggest that it is associated with a reduced daily caloric intake. If you haven't already, read Chapter 4 for the real skinny on breakfast.

"**I'm afraid I'll get too tired and hungry.**" Again, you may have to try this to believe it, but most people adapt well to this regimen. Because it keeps your energy level up and your appetite down, excessive fatigue or hunger is rarely an issue. You may actually find yourself feeling less tired and hungry than you do after eating cereal, toast, or other typical breakfast items. For additional suggestions, read the section "Tame the Raging Appetite" in the next chapter.

Let's say that you follow this program, do everything right, and you're still hungry. Then eat! Try it again the next day and see if you do better. Should you discover that you really do need to eat more often during the day, try to wait at least 2 hours after eating before you exercise, and refrain from eating for as long as possible afterward. This will give you the best chances of turning on and remaining in the fat-burning mode.

"**I don't have time to exercise in the morning.**" Now, this is a valid concern. Morning exercise is hard for many people. Having small children at home, an early workday, school, a long commute, a nocturnal lifestyle, or other factors can certainly complicate morning schedules, but there are ways to fit it in. In the section in the next chapter entitled "Time Won't Let Me . . . ," I've made a number of suggestions for solving this dilemma. However, if you really are unable to exercise in the morning, you may opt for the afternoon or evening exercise options discussed later in this chapter.

"I'm not sure if I can exercise five times a week." The mini-fast is not an all-or-nothing proposal, and no one is perfect 100 percent of the time. If you can manage to fit in exercise 4, 3, or occasionally just 2 days a week—and you clean up your diet—you can expect to see results. Do your best and be as consistent as possible. Although your progress may be slower, it is likely that you will still lose weight.

"My schedule is unpredictable—I can't fast and exercise at the same time every day." You don't have to. Flexibility is fine. For example, if you've opted for morning exercise but miss a session due to an early meeting, skip lunch and take a walk during that time. Or if you usually fast and work out in the evenings but have dinner plans, simply modify your schedule. The goal is to exercise in the fasting state. Precisely when is less important.

"I don't want to give up my favorite foods." You don't have to. Although I've provided food suggestions, recipes, and menu plans in Chapters 11 and 12, this is not a restricted diet. If your favorite foods are brownies and onion rings, you may have to eat them sparingly and make concessions in other areas. But no single food is off-limits.

"I've never been successful on any diet before, and even if I lose weight, I always gain it back." The mini-fast with exercise incorporates the essential ingredient for weight loss—fat burning—in a program that does not require extreme dieting or food restrictions. I am not saying it's easy. You're going to have to discipline yourself to put on your walking shoes a few times a week and exert some control over your caloric intake. But exercising in the fasting state curbs appetite and accelerates fat burning like nothing else. And keep in mind that this is not a short-term diet but a lifestyle that will help keep you slim and healthy for years to come.

"I don't have much self-discipline, and I'm not sure I can stick with this program." I don't have much self-discipline either. Few people do. Unfortunately, you and you alone have to make the decision to do something about your weight, then muster the will and the self-control to do it. I've included a section in the next chapter called "Motivate Yourself with Instant Willpower." It describes a system that I and many of my patients have used to change behaviors and adopt health-promoting habits. In a nutshell, you make a signed contract with yourself that has an unpleasant consequence—such as writing a check to an organization you intensely dislike—in the event that you fail to follow through on your commitment. You have to be willing to actually pony up, but it is an extremely powerful motivator. In Chapter 6, I've also provided a few other suggestions to help you find the resolve and determination to stick with this program.

"I go to bed early. Does the same time frame apply to me?" Early to bed, early to rise—and early to exercise? By all means, don't feel like you have to wait until noon to eat. The mini-fast with exercise hinges upon the concept of maintaining fat burning for a protracted period. It begins with aerobic exercise while fasting and ends with eating. If you exercise at 5:00 a.m., of course you can eat before noon. You'll already have been burning fat for hours.

"I'm an intense exerciser. I'm worried about losing muscle if I don't get any protein in the morning." This is another very valid consideration, which came from one of my newsletter subscribers. The mini-fast with exercise is designed for overweight people, most of whom are not intense exercisers. The most popular type of exercise is brisk walking. Protein supplementation is not necessary with this moderate degree of exercise. However, it may well be for athletic individuals who exercise more vigorously. If you fall into this category, having a protein drink before you exercise is a good idea. Aim for 10 to 20 grams of protein and around 100 calories, and no more than 10 to 12 grams of carbohydrates.

"I'm not sure about the supplements." Then don't take them. The supplements created for the mini-fast with exercise are completely optional. As I've said, some people swear by them, while others don't think they make a whit of difference and do perfectly fine without them. They are an adjunct to the program, not a requirement.

"I like the idea, but I'm in such bad shape I really can't exercise." Building up to the recommended exercise duration and intensity must be done gradually. Most anybody can go for a short walk, and that's good enough for starters. If you have arthritis or another condition that prohibits weight-bearing activities, then consider swimming or riding a stationary bike. Regardless, get clearance from your physician before beginning this or any other exercise program if you are in poor condition or have any serious medical problems.

"I have type 2 diabetes. Can I do the mini-fast with exercise?" We "prescribe" the mini-fast with exercise to virtually every patient with type 2 diabetes who comes through the doors of the Whitaker Wellness Institute. This program is tailor-made for them. As they lose weight, they experience dramatic improvements in insulin sensitivity, blood sugar control, medication requirements, complications of diabetes, and overall health and wellbeing. I want to note that patients with type 2 diabetes, especially those who are taking insulin or sulfonylurea (medications that stimulate insulin secretion), should talk to their doctors before beginning this regimen. It's possible that they may experience a hypoglycemic reaction—blood sugar may go too low. Anyone with diabetes should monitor his or her blood sugar level when starting the mini-fast with exercise program; it has an ameliorating effect on blood sugar levels, and, under a physician's supervision, medication usage may need to be modified.

"I don't know if my doctor will be supportive." I guarantee that your doctor will be supportive of weight loss. The mini-fast with exercise has been around for 15 years, but many physicians are unfamiliar with it. Most will be on board with the exercise and calorie restriction, but skipping breakfast could be outside their comfort zone. This book contains more than 150 scientific references, many of them directly in support of various aspects of the program. I also have considerable clinical experience under my belt, and hundreds of patients under the care of the Whitaker Wellness Institute are currently on the program. Most of these patients are also dealing with type 2 diabetes, coronary artery disease, metabolic syndrome, and other serious health problems. Across the board they are tolerating the program well, losing weight, and experiencing improvements in blood sugar, lipids, blood pressure, energy, and more. In the unlikely event that your doctor dismisses the mini-fast with exercise outright, I suggest that you get a second opinion from a more open-minded physician. Weight loss is far too important to let one person's uninformed opinion prevent you from taking advantage of this very effective program and its multiple health benefits.

ON YOUR MARK, GET SET . . .

You now have all the knowledge and the tools required for success on the mini-fast with exercise. For those of you who would like additional information and guidance, it's all here in this book. In

CHECKLIST FOR GETTING STARTED

✔ Select a date to begin and commit to sticking with the program for a designated period of time, say, 3 or 4 weeks for starters.

✔ Decide on the particulars, i.e., time and days to exercise, and prioritize them by scheduling them into your calendar.

✔ Get clearance from your doctor if you have a serious medical condition.

✔ Order optional supplements if you plan to use them. (www.drwhitaker.com; 800-722-8008)

✔ Track your progress by recording baseline information such as weight, hip and waist circumference, etc. (See Chapter 7 for details and forms.)

✔ Set your alarm to wake up in the morning and begin your journey to leanness and optimal health.

the next four chapters, I have provided a number of suggestions for staying on track, assessing your current status, monitoring your progress, and addressing medical issues that may be holding you back. Part III: Exercise and Diet Strategies details a walking program as well as a progressive wogging regimen and strength-training exercises that you can do at home. It also includes the diet recommendations that we give our patients at Whitaker Wellness, a 2-week meal plan, and delicious recipes created especially for the Mini-Fast Diet by the nutritionists and professional chefs at the Rodale Test Kitchen.

Beyond that, the only things missing are your desire, resolve, and commitment to make the lifestyle changes necessary for weight loss. Once you get started, you will be pleasantly surprised at how energetic and hunger free you feel during your mini-fasts. You will marvel at the ease with which you are able to reduce your daily caloric intake, not by starving yourself but simply by skipping breakfast and eating healthy foods. Best of all, you will experience the inevitable weight loss—specifically, fat loss—that comes when you're vigorously burning fat on the Mini-Fast Diet.

Steve: "Stay Focused on My Goal"

Steve, a patient from Laughlin, Nevada, is both camera- and publicity-shy. Although I can't share his photos, I can tell you that he's looking and feeling great—and he's sold on the Mini-Fast Diet. Here is his story.

"I have been overweight for at least 10 years, and at my heaviest I was carrying around 50 excess pounds. I've never had much success with any other program, and I've tried everything from a healthy breakfast to eating just protein. I once lost 25 pounds after a trip to India, but that was unintentional and I wouldn't recommend that 'diet' to anyone. I started the mini-fast with exercise because my doctor at Whitaker Wellness told me that I needed to lose weight. At that point I weighed 250 pounds, felt tired all the time, and knew that the extra weight wasn't doing my knees any good.

"This program is much easier than I would have expected. Skipping breakfast isn't hard, and I am not at all hungry in the mornings. I also increased my exercise. I used to walk maybe ½ mile 3 days a week, but I increased this to 4 miles, which takes about an hour, and I do it almost every day.

"Since I began this program 5 months ago, I have lost 25 pounds and 4 inches off my waist. I now weigh 225. My goal is 200 pounds, but even after I reach it, I plan to make this regimen a permanent part of my life. With other programs I was always hungry. The advantage of the mini-fast is that I feel like my body has easily adjusted to not eating until lunchtime.

"When I first started, I lost weight rapidly because I also significantly cut calories. Then I began to get bored—like I always did on other diets—and started eating desserts, etc. Now I am back to eating regular, full meals, but they are much healthier. I cut back on bread, potatoes, and sugar and eat a lot of steamed vegetables and meat. I am not a cook and I eat out a lot, but I have learned that you can order healthy foods in restaurants. I also have protein drinks regularly, and I take Dr. Whitaker's supplements, which are very helpful.

"I still have some issues with portion control, but I follow the program religiously, check my weight daily, and stay focused on my goal."

CHAPTER 6

STAYING ON TRACK

Success is not final, failure is not fatal: It is the courage to continue that counts.

—WINSTON CHURCHILL

Getting started on the mini-fast with exercise is just the beginning. Staying on track and sticking with the program is what really matters. Surveys suggest that the average dieter makes four weight loss attempts per year.[1] That doesn't speak well for either the success of most approaches out there or the tenacity of most dieters. I'm not going to tell you that the mini-fast with exercise is effortless or guarantee that you'll lose weight. Anyone who promises easy, surefire weight loss is just not being honest.

This program, like any sustainable weight loss program, requires making lifestyle changes, which, as everyone knows, is no piece of cake. Any type of change requires determination and a willingness to get outside your comfort zone, and these things come easier for some people than for others. Eliminating breakfast (or another meal) will probably take some getting used to, and although that step alone may well be enough of a caloric reduction, if you are a big eater and your diet includes lots of fats, sugars, and unhealthy foods, you must make adjustments in these areas as well. The other requirement is that you have to exercise. The exercise itself is not overly strenuous or time-consuming, but you must fit it into your schedule and keep it up on a regular basis. If you do put in the effort to make these changes, the end result—a slimmer body and better health—is well within your grasp.

So how can you make this endeavor different? How can you ensure that this time you really will muster the resolve to stay the course? In this chapter I'm going to address the two most common pitfalls of all weight loss programs: making the time to exercise and taming a raging appetite. I'll also tell you about "instant will-power," my exceptionally effective technique for self-discipline and motivation, along with other strategies that have been helpful for my patients and others who have made the mini-fast with exercise part of their permanent daily routine.

"TIME WON'T LET ME . . ."

The exercise requirement for this program is moderate aerobic activity for 30 to 60 minutes 3 to 5 days a week, and the most popular activity is brisk walking. Provided that you don't have a serious medical problem, this type of physical activity is eminently doable. For most of us, however, our ability to exercise is not the hang-up. Making exercise a priority and fitting it into an already busy schedule can be a bear—and are among the most frequent objections I hear regarding this program. Exercise seems to be the first activity that people jettison when they're crunched for time.

This really doesn't make sense. We're talking only an average of 45 minutes 4 days a week: That's 3 hours a week. I would be willing to bet that you spend far more time than that watching TV or updating your Facebook page. Three hours a week shouldn't be that daunting, especially for something as health-affirming, mood-boosting, and ego-empowering as exercise.

Morning exercise can be doubly challenging. Most workplaces require employees to show up at a relatively early hour, and some of you may have a long commute on top of that. If you have children, mornings are even more hectic. In addition, those who characterize themselves as night owls just have a hard time getting going in the mornings. So what do you do?

- **Get up earlier.** The most obvious solution is to reset your alarm clock and get up earlier in the morning. If that means going to bed earlier, so be it.

- **Restructure your routine.** Some of us rise early but still manage to fritter away the morning reading the paper, checking e-mail, drinking coffee, and preparing and/or eating breakfast. I'm not sure how it happens, but some mornings I'll look at the clock and realize that I've been awake for 3 hours with nothing to show for it. The solution here is to prioritize exercise and do it before settling into your morning routine.

- **Make your mornings less hectic.** My children are all college-age or older now, but I certainly recall the chaos of getting a houseful of kids ready for school and out the door in the morning. Organizing things the night before—laying out clothes, putting homework in backpacks, and making lunches, for example—will free up time the following day. Even if there are no kids in the picture, taking care of business before you go to bed makes mornings more relaxed and opens up time for exercise.

- **Exercise after the hustle and bustle die down.** Nobody says you have to bounce out of bed and exercise. You could take an early break and walk after you get to work, if your schedule allows, or exercise after you see the kids off. Small children can be bundled up and taken with you in a stroller or a bike seat, and older ones can ride, walk, or jog alongside you. A friend of mine who babysits for her son and daughter-in-law 1 day a week simply carries her granddaughter as she walks briskly around the neighborhood. She told me that her arms have become noticeably stronger and her endurance greater as the baby has gotten bigger over the course of a year.

- **Get some help.** If you are married with kids, have his and hers mornings—one day it's your turn to take care of the morning craziness, and the next day it's your spouse's turn so you can exercise. Trading off babysitting duties a few mornings a week with another parent might also work. And remember that some gyms and exercise facilities offer child care.

There are only 24 hours in a day, and if you truly can't fit in morning exercise, you will have to consider another option—skipping lunch or dinner and working out during that time. To learn more about these and other options for personalizing the mini-fast with exercise, see Chapter 5.

TAME THE RAGING APPETITE

A voracious appetite can booby-trap any weight loss program. As I've mentioned, we are hardwired to eat to our heart's content when food is plentiful. It's a survival tool, an outgrowth of the feast-or-famine conditions in which our ancestors evolved—get your fill today in case there's nothing to eat tomorrow. For most of you reading this, food is *too* readily available. It's perpetual feast time, and this is a primary reason why we gain weight and most diets fail. Our natural instincts make it hard for us to say no to food.

The mini-fast with exercise does a decent job of taming appetite while restricting calories. What else, besides skipping a meal, allows you to significantly reduce your daily caloric intake without counting calories or making adjustments throughout the day? As long as you don't make up for it by stuffing yourself after noon, skipping breakfast will lead to weight loss. In the event that you do find yourself hungry—if you can't wait until lunch to eat or you cannot help but overeat the rest of the day—then what? Here are some tips that might help.

- **Exercise in the fasting state.** On the days that you exercise while mini-fasting, you're going to feel less hungry. Exercise rapidly uses up the glycogen stores that have been fueling your body since your last meal and kicks you into fat-burning mode. When fat is used for energy, ketones are produced as a by-product, and this state, called ketosis, blunts appetite. The hunger-dulling aspect of ketosis is another evolutionary "trick" that makes fasting more comfortable. If you are unbearably hungry on your days off, try some of the following suggestions—or exercise. Moderate aerobic exercise isn't so strenuous that you can't do it most days of the week.

- **Have a cup of coffee, tea, or other calorie-free drink.** Coffee is my go-to beverage when I feel like eating in the morning. Caffeine perks you up and makes you feel better and more alert. It also has a slight appetite-suppressing effect that will help you get through the fasting period. In addition, it stimulates fat burning, again to a fairly minor degree, but every little bit helps. Finally, it gives you something to do with your hands and put in your mouth. Like a smoker who is trying to quit, one of the most difficult things about skipping meals is finding a replacement activity. For me and for many of my patients, having a cup or two of coffee or tea—or any other noncaloric beverage—fills that need and takes the edge off. Feel free to use a calorie-free sweetener (stevia and xylitol are my favorites), and a little creamer won't hurt. But stay away from sugary, carbohydrate-rich, flavored coffee drinks. They will stop fat burning in its tracks.

- **Avoid foods that cause blood sugar swings.** The diet recommendations in Chapters 11 and 12 are foods that fill you up and tide you over. Sweets, potatoes, bread, pasta, and most everything made with sugar or refined grains—think white foods—have a high glycemic index and load. This means they rapidly drive up blood glucose but may be followed a couple of hours later by reactive hypoglycemia, a compensatory blood sugar dive that makes you tired, sluggish, and so hungry you feel like you could eat a cow. These crashes can easily sabotage any diet. To avoid this very common phenomenon, eat more fiber-rich vegetables and beans and include some protein with every meal. These foods are not only bulky, filling, and lower in calories, but because they cause a gradual rise in blood sugar, they will keep you going longer and are less apt to stimulate food cravings.

- **Have a snack.** If you are hungry between meals outside your mini-fasting period (for the majority of people, this means in the afternoon), by all means, eat something. Snacking is actually encouraged on this program. We don't want you to feel deprived, plus snacking reduces your odds of overeating at dinner. Just make sure that the foods you select are healthy, and be particularly wary of high-glycemic snacks that perpetuate blood sugar swings. Try one of these patient favorites that can be eaten on the go: a handful of nuts, a piece of string cheese, or half of a meal-replacement bar or drink. For more suggestions, see Chapter 11.

♦ **Beware of mindless eating.** My wife and I were recently eating out with another couple and had just completed a great meal. We all had plenty to eat and were perfectly full when the waiter came by with dessert menus. All of a sudden, four people who had declared themselves stuffed minutes earlier were debating what to order for dessert. Most of us have had the experience of eating when we're not hungry. We may be bored, stressed, or merely in the presence of a favorite item. Or we could be watching TV, reading, or otherwise focused on something else and eating more or less unconsciously. That's the power that food can have over us. Be aware of these traps and of the propensity for mindless eating, and do your best to avoid it.

♦ **Take supplements that curb appetite.** I've told you about the nutritional supplements that many of my patients take before exercising and during the mini-fasting period to reduce appetite, and I'll discuss others in later chapters. (I won't go into detail here, other than to refer you to the list in "Supplements to Take the Edge Off.") If an out-of-control appetite and overeating are waylaying your weight loss efforts, I strongly suggest that you give one or more of these safe, natural supplements a try.

♦ **If all else fails, go ahead and eat before noon.** There's no magic about 12:00 noon. The only reason I suggest waiting until then to eat is because that's when most people eat lunch. Let's say that it's 10:30 or 11:00 a.m., and all you can think about is food. Go ahead and eat. Breaking your fast a little early isn't going to derail your weight loss. Just remember that the longer you wait to eat after exercising, the longer you will be in a fat-burning state.

SUPPLEMENTS TO TAKE THE EDGE OFF

Optional nutritional supplements that I recommend as part of the Mini-Fast Diet include a few amino acids and herbal extracts that directly affect appetite. I discuss them in greater detail elsewhere in this book, but here they are in brief.

Ketosis Essentials is specially formulated to make the mini-fast with exercise more comfortable by staving off the low energy, irritable mood, and hunger that may come with fasting. The combination of hydroxycitric acid (HCA),[2] L-carnitine, glycine, and chromium has a synergy that reduces appetite, enhances fat burning, and improves exercise endurance. The suggested dose is one scoop mixed in water before exercise and a second during the post-exercise fasting period, if hunger is an issue.[3]

Metabolic Essentials is a proprietary blend of a standardized green tea extract called GreenSelect Phytosome, other botanicals, magnesium, and vitamin D. In addition to helping with appetite, this supplement targets multiple aspects of metabolic syndrome.[4] To use, take two capsules twice a day, with lunch and dinner.

5-hydroxytryptophan (5-HTP) is a precursor to serotonin, a neurotransmitter that improves mood, helps curb appetite, and reduces carbohydrate cravings.[5] The starting dosage is 50 milligrams 20 minutes before lunch and dinner and may be increased to 100 milligrams, taken up to three times a day.

Saffron is an herbal extract that also increases serotonin levels. In studies, a standardized saffron extract called Satiereal has been shown to reduce stress eating and between-meals snacking.[6] The dose used in this research was 90 milligrams twice a day.

GET BY WITH A LITTLE HELP FROM YOUR FRIENDS

In addition to the suggestions we've covered so far for sticking with the mini-fast with exercise program, do not overlook or neglect to ask for help from your family and friends. There's nothing like the support of others to keep you on track with any positive lifestyle change. If you want to stop smoking, get off drugs or alcohol, work out, or follow a diet, having a cheerleader or a comrade in arms can make the path smoother and the goal closer.

Some people are fortunate enough to be married to their "support group." Ken Wright, a patient at Whitaker Wellness, is a perfect example. Ken was in terrible shape. Morbidly obese at 444 pounds, he had diabetes with almost every complication imaginable, including neuropathy and retinopathy. He had such severe pain in his legs that he was unable to walk and had to get around in a motorized wheelchair. It was Ken's wife, Mourlene, a subscriber to my newsletter, who insisted that he come to the clinic (Ken had initially dismissed us as "a bunch of quacks"). But after his doctors at home told him there was nothing else they could do for him, Mourlene put her foot down.

So they came to Whitaker Wellness and stayed for 2 weeks. Ken was treated with a number of therapies to get his diabetes and pain under control, and they both attended our educational program of lectures and personalized instruction in diet, exercise, and other lifestyle changes. Then they went home and got down to the business of implementing these changes. A year and 2 months later, Ken had lost 165 pounds and 20 inches around his waist. He discontinued 10 of the 13 drugs he had been on, and was exercising regularly, eating right (thanks to Mourlene), and feeling better than he had in 20 years.

We see the importance of support like this at the clinic all the time. Most often it's a spouse—who in some cases drags the other in kicking and screaming. But it can also be a parent or an adult child, a brother or sister, or a good friend who initiates and facilitates the journey back to health. Take advantage of the people in your life who care about you. Nobody likes to be the nagger or the "naggee," but most everybody can use a swift kick in the pants from time to time, particularly if it involves issues as important as weight and health.

Find or Start a Support Group

It's an unfortunate fact of life that not everyone has a built-in support group. If you don't, find a local group or create one of your own. You could become a member of an organization like Weight Watchers. The weekly meetings and weigh-ins required by this and similar programs are largely responsible for their success. You'll get to spend time with like-minded people who'll offer support and encouragement. Furthermore, you will get recognition for your efforts and accomplishments, which can be highly motivating. (One word of caution: These programs will probably suggest that you eat breakfast. Pay attention to their general recommendations, but ignore this advice.)

In addition to support groups that specifically target weight loss, I suggest that you consider organized exercise programs. Personal trainers are excellent, as are all types of exercise classes. Although they can be pricey, simply paying for a gym membership or a series of classes is often enough to get you off your duff and into the gym. And if you take regularly scheduled classes, you're more likely to get into the groove of showing up at a given hour on certain days of the week. Other options include signing up for tennis, racquetball, or squash "ladders," which pair you with other players, or joining a cycling or running club. You'll enjoy the camaraderie *and* you'll become more active.

Not much of a joiner? Then enlist a friend or a co-worker to exercise with you. You're much less likely to blow off a scheduled activity if it means standing up this person. I always get a kick out of seeing two of the women who work at Whitaker Wellness striding around the block at a good clip in their work clothes and running shoes. They tell me that they do this several days a week in place of their lunch breaks, and in addition to the exercise, it gives them a chance to chat.

Is Obesity Contagious?

There's something to be said for hanging out with people who share your desires for health and fitness. In fact, a growing number of studies suggest that obesity is contagious—it spreads through social networks like sniffles and coughs during the cold and flu season. If a close friend or a family member gains a lot of weight, your risk of doing the same dramatically increases. I'm not saying that obesity is caused by a virus or other infectious disease. Rather, it is the *acceptability* of obesity that appears to be communicable. When people we care about get fat, it becomes less of a stigma for us to follow suit. Being overweight becomes more than okay; it becomes the new social norm.

In a landmark study published in the *New England Journal of Medicine,* Harvard researchers looked at the links between obesity and social circles, or networks. This study involved more than 12,000 people who were enrolled in the long-term and ongoing Framingham Heart Study. For a 32-year period between 1971 and 2003, they were regularly reevaluated and their weight, BMI, and other health markers were tracked. Because the Framingham Study is centralized to one town in Massachusetts and is now in its third generation—it began in 1948, and these participants are offspring of the original study subjects—there were tens of thousands of social and family ties within this group. Nearly half had a friend in the network, 83 percent had a spouse in it, and 87 percent had a sibling in the group. The study subjects also provided information about other family members and close friends.

The researchers found that social networks have a very powerful influence on weight. If a friend became obese, an individual's chances of also becoming obese increased by 57 percent. And if the friend was a close one, the risk ballooned to 171 percent. The trend was strongest among male friendships. Somewhat weaker yet still significant associations were noted among girlfriends, spouses, and siblings of both sexes. But it had to be a reasonably close tie rather than a casual acquaintance. Immediate neighbors, for example, did not affect one another's weight, but good friends and family members who lived at a distance did.[7]

Weight Loss and Healthy Habits Are Also Contagious

If obesity in those who are near and dear to us increases our chances of gaining weight, could the opposite also be true? Are weight loss and positive, healthy habits and lifestyle changes also contagious? The authors of the Harvard study believe so.

> The spread of obesity in social networks appears to be a factor in the obesity epidemic. Yet the relevance of social influence also suggests that it may be possible to harness this same force to slow the spread of obesity. Network phenomena might be exploited to spread positive health behaviors, in part because people's perceptions of their own risk of illness may depend on the people around them. . . . People are connected, and so their health is connected.[8]

To test this premise and see if weight loss also had a "ripple effect" and would spread through social networks, a research team at the University of Connecticut enrolled the spouses of participants in a placebo-controlled clinical trial evaluating the effects of weight loss on cardiovascular disease in overweight people with type 2 diabetes. The participants in the original study were randomly assigned to one of two groups: an intensive lifestyle intervention program or enhanced usual care, essentially a placebo group.

The 357 spouses in the "ripple effect study" were not part of the weight loss trial. They were simply married to, living, dining, and interacting with, and presumably being influenced by those who were. This study showed that weight loss is also communicable. The spouses of the subjects assigned to the intensive lifestyle intervention group lost an average of 4.8 pounds over the course of a year, and 26 percent of them lost at least 5 percent of their total body weight. In comparison, individuals married to those in the placebo group lost less than half a pound, and just 9 percent reduced their weight by 5 percent.[9]

You've probably seen similar effects in your own social circles. I know I have. A few years ago, one of my staff members was determined to lose 30 pounds before her wedding. Months before the big day, she began exercising in earnest and cutting back on her caloric intake. Rather than going out for lunch, she brought in healthy leftovers and ate in the office. Not only did this woman drop those 30 pounds, but her co-worker, who usually had lunch with her, also lost weight.

I've experienced this phenomenon personally. My wife, Connie, is an exercise maniac. In addition to working out with a personal trainer twice a week, she "wogs" (walks and jogs) on streets and trails near the house with me 2 or 3 days a week. Doing it together certainly makes me more compliant. There are days I'd rather sleep in or drink coffee and read the newspaper. But knowing that my own "personal trainer" is waiting for me at the front door gets me moving.

THE MINI-FAST IS "INFECTIOUS"

I can tell you for a fact that the mini-fast with exercise is contagious. When we conducted our 12-week study on this protocol at the clinic, the first people we invited to participate were our employees. We asked them up front for two reasons. First, they didn't require a big outside recruitment effort, and, second, we knew where to find them so we could stalk them if they didn't follow up.

Talk about a domino effect! Not only did we have a tremendous amount of interest among people who work at the clinic, but they told their friends and family members about it. Before we knew it, our phones were ringing off the hook. We had kids and spouses, sisters and brothers, mothers-in-law and uncles, neighbors and friends from the gym, even a waiter at a restaurant near the clinic and his daughter wanted to participate. Not everyone qualified, but word of mouth spread so rapidly and so far that we had to cut off enrollment. One of our longtime employees told her daughter about the mini-fast. Her daughter told a friend, who told a friend, who told another friend. I believe that six people got involved and lost weight all because of one person.

This is a clear illustration of the power of social networks on positive health behaviors. The mini-fast with exercise is new. It's different and exciting and it works. Use this to your advantage by passing the information in this book on to the people in your social circles and encouraging them to join you in adopting a healthy lifestyle and achieving permanent weight control.

MOTIVATE YOURSELF WITH INSTANT WILLPOWER

I have one additional suggestion for those of you who are having a hard time getting started or staying on the program. Wanting to make the requisite lifestyle changes isn't enough. The way that most people go about such desires is the same way they make New Year's resolutions—with vague plans and promises to do this or not do that. Let's take the perennial favorite, "I'm going to start exercising," which is certainly appropriate for this discussion. Exercise is a worthy, achievable goal, and many people start the year off with a bang. Health clubs and exercise classes are notoriously crowded in January; by March, attendance is back to normal. Why? Because changing personal habits requires focus, effort, and discipline. It requires willpower.

The Mini-Fast Diet, like any weight loss regimen, requires willpower, no doubt about it. Unfortunately, many of us think of ourselves as being rather short in that department; we believe self-discipline and resolve are not our strong suit. But let me remind you that, in some areas of your life, you are highly disciplined. Most of you have or have had a job at one time or another. Most jobs have a starting time, say 8:30 a.m. So you get there every day by 8:30 because you know that if you didn't, there would be hell to pay. Imagine if you decided to arrive whenever you felt like it, showing up at 9:15 one day and 10:00 the next. There would be a well-defined consequence—you'd get fired.

We do many things in our lives because we're afraid of the consequences if we don't do them. We pay our taxes, a decidedly unpleasant task, because we know that we could get in big trouble if we didn't. For similar reasons, we drive close to the speed limit and pay our rent or mortgage payment on time. Fear of consequences is a very powerful motivator. What are the consequences of overeating and sitting on the couch? Getting fat and unhealthy, right? And although I don't know anyone who actually enjoys being heavy or sick, this obviously isn't enough of an incentive for the two-thirds of Americans who are overweight. If it were, we wouldn't be having this discussion.

Now I want to show you how to harness the same degree of motivation that makes you get to work on time in order to help you develop healthy habits and achieve your weight loss goals. It's a technique I've employed numerous times myself—usually with success—and one I encourage my patients to use. I call it instant willpower. All you have to do is create consequences that, like getting fired, going to jail, or losing your home, will essentially force you to take action. Then, to keep yourself on the up-and-up, you need to put the lifestyle changes you want to make and the consequences you're willing to pay, should you not fulfill your end of the bargain, in a contract, sign it, have it witnessed, and treat it like any other binding agreement. Let's use exercise as an example. Here's what you do.

1. Select the type of exercise, the number of times a week you want to do it, and the length of each session. For example, let's say that you want to walk 4 days a week for 45 minutes at a time. This is a great goal. It's specific and it's achievable. Most people are physically capable of walking and can squeeze in 45 minutes of exercise four times a week.

2. Decide on the duration of your contract. Limit it to a length of time that you know you can accomplish. Don't, for instance, make a promise for a year, as this substantially decreases your chances of success. Three weeks or a month is a manageable period, and if it goes well, you can extend the contract.

3. Come up with a consequence that you will have to live with if you fail to exercise, per your contract. The most effective consequences, in my opinion, are monetary. Everyone hates to part with a buck, so pledge to give a certain amount of money to an institution or entity that you *don't* want to give money to. Promising $100 to your children's college fund, your church, or your favorite charity won't work. Select an organization that you *dis*like. If you're a staunch Democrat, it could be a donation to the National Republican Committee. If you're a Republican, it could be to the National Democratic Committee. If you're apolitical, then find something else that's particularly odious to you. The goal is to make it painful, but

realistic. Obviously, a very large payment is a greater incentive. However, if you do this on a frequent basis, as I have over the past 15 years, there will be times when you fail to follow through on your commitment and must pay up. Therefore, it's important that your pledge be within your means. You must be willing and able to write that check if you fall off the wagon. If you aren't, then why bother?

4. Write up a contract similar to the form below, sign and date it, and have it witnessed. This step is very important. Breaking a promise to yourself is easy—we do it all the time. But when others are involved, it ups the ante. Post your signed contract in a prominent place where you'll be reminded of it. And if you really want to make it stick, tell your friends, family, and co-workers what you're doing. This means that, in addition to the financial consequences, you will have to face a little public embarrassment if you flake out.

INSTANT WILLPOWER CONTRACT

I _____ agree to _____

for _____ beginning _____.

If I so much as _____

I agree to give $_____ to _____.

Signed _____

Witnessed by _____ Date _____

My Personal Example

Let me tell you about one of the first times I made such a contract and what I learned from it. I wanted to lose 20 pounds, so I pledged to do just that in 2½ months. My consequence, if I were to fail, was to send $10,000 to the Bill Clinton Legal Defense Fund. (This was during the days of the Monica Lewinsky affair, and I wasn't a big fan of Clinton anyway, so this seemed as reasonable a consequence as any.) Then I wrote about it in my newsletter, *Health & Healing,* which went out to hundreds of thousands of subscribers.

No sooner had the newsletter gone to press than it dawned on me what I'd done. You can bet on outcomes in Vegas and your fantasy sports leagues, but weight loss isn't as clear-cut. Even if you are thoroughly committed to doing all the work—in the case of the mini-fast, skipping breakfast and exercising regularly—there is no guarantee that you will lose a specific number of pounds in a given period of time. Instant willpower contracts should never be about outcomes. They should be about behaviors that are within your control, such as the activities you do or do not do or the specific foods you eat or do not eat. Nevertheless, the die was cast, and there was no turning back. Everybody knew about my contract.

I think I worked out harder and ate less during that period than at any other time in my life. As a man of my word, I was willing to honor my pledge, and $10K is a big chunk of change. That's another lesson I learned from this experience—make the amount realistic. Don't go betting $1,000 if $100 is a stretch for you. But the most important lesson I learned was the value of making the contracts public. The idea of having to tell everyone around the clinic, not to mention all those *Health & Healing* readers, that I had failed was actually more painful than the thought of writing that check. I was sweating bullets for 2 months, but I squeaked by with a few days to spare. My subsequent contracts have been for behaviors, not outcomes. They've also been for shorter periods of time and less significant sums of money. But I continue to use instant willpower contracts, and I suggest that you try it yourself.

No one is going to fire you if you don't stick with this program. You're not going to get a ticket or go to jail. Your friends and family aren't going to look down on you. In fact, most likely, nobody is even going to know that you tried and failed to follow a weight loss program. That's why it's so easy to give up after a few days, stop exercising, and go back to eating bagels for breakfast. There are no consequences. Instant willpower contracts simply increase your personal accountability.

IT'S TIME TO GET SERIOUS ABOUT WEIGHT LOSS

If you really want to make a success of this, you'll need to pull out all the stops. Sit down with your calendar or planner and find a space for exercise in your schedule, using some of my suggestions for working through the usual issues that make mornings a challenge. Decide on specific times, dates, and activities, and treat your exercise sessions as you would any other important appointment. Take a hard look at your diet. Skipping breakfast may be the extent of the changes you need to make in this area, but be realistic. If your diet requires an overall tune-up, now is the time to make improvements. And if overeating and hunger are driving you off course, try some of the solutions discussed in this chapter that have worked for others.

Enlist the support of your family, friends, and others, and accept any and all help you can get. To improve compliance, make

an "instant willpower" contract with yourself, and use the tracking form in the next chapter to monitor your progress. You may
fall off the wagon—it happens to the best of us. If you do, get up,
brush yourself off, and start again.

Achieving your optimal weight, feeling good about yourself,
and looking great to others will be worth every hour you exercise,
every cinnamon roll you pass up, and every other effort you make
to solve your weight problem once and for all.

MINI-FAST DIET *Success Story*

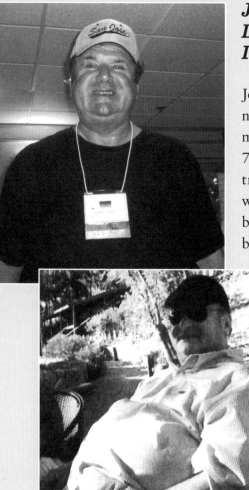

John Sorci at 360 pounds, before the Mini-Fast Diet, and after (top)

John Sorci: "I Plan to Do This for as Long as I Live"

John Sorci, from San Jose, California, had tremendous success on the mini-fast with exercise—he lost 70 pounds in a year—but he got off track and regained some of the weight. Once he realized how much better he felt on the program, he got back in gear and is now committed and determined to stay the course. I'm sharing John's story as an inspiration for those of you who have also strayed off the path and want to find it again. Just do what John did: Pick up the pieces and start over.

"I never had much of a weight problem until my forties, when I started putting on a few extra pounds, but the weight gain really picked up after I retired. I also developed a lot of health problems around that time, including type 2 diabetes, hypertension, high cholesterol and triglycerides, and heart problems. I had little energy and a lot of back pain as well. I've always known that part of my problem was my weight, and I also didn't like the way I looked.

But I just could not seem to get my weight down. I tried Weight Watchers, which was too tedious, and Jenny Craig, but I wasn't crazy about the food.

"I heard about the mini-fast with exercise from my doctor at the Whitaker Wellness Institute, where I have been going for 2 years. Even though it is quite a distance from my home, this clinic has helped me so much that it is worth the trip down to Newport Beach. When my doctor suggested that I try the mini-fast, I thought, 'Why not?'

"When I first began, I weighed 360 pounds. I started exercising, and I changed my diet and ate more salads and vegetables. Because I live alone and am not much of a cook, I also ordered food from a company that prepares meals and delivers them to my home. For snacks, I had protein shakes. In approximately 1 year, I lost 70 pounds, and my pants size decreased by 10 inches. I was very pleased with myself. My blood sugar and blood pressure went down, my blood work improved, and I had less sciatic pain in my hip because I had less weight to carry around.

"I hate to admit it, but I fell off the wagon. I got lax with my exercise and diet. I began eating out more and more—not fast food, but restaurants can be just as bad. And I gained some of that weight back. I finally decided no more, and I got back on the mini-fast. Now I walk almost every day, and I also use a treadmill and small weights. I'm skipping breakfast again, which was a little different the first time, but it's easy to get used to. I do not get hungry, and this gives me a great sense of control. I also take a lot of nutritional supplements, for my medical conditions as well as the specific supplements Dr. Whitaker recommends for the mini-fast, and they help a lot.

"I now feel healthier, livelier, and have much more energy. On a scale of 1 to 10, I used to be a 2. Now I'm a 7. I know I'm going to have to keep myself motivated, but knowing what happened when I stopped the program is enough motivation for me. My goal is to get back down to 220 pounds, which I know I can do because I did it before. Once I get there, I plan to keep it up. I will be doing the mini-fast for as long as I live!"

CHAPTER 7

MONITORING YOUR PROGRESS

Marge, the bathroom scale is lying again!

—HOMER SIMPSON

Nobody wants to be heavy. Unless you're a sumo wrestler, it's not something you strive for. I don't know anyone who made a conscious decision to get fat, but for two out of every three people in the United States, it happened. Because weight gain is intimately linked to habits related to food and activity, it's to some degree unconscious. (A habit by definition is "a recurrent, often unconscious pattern of behavior acquired through frequent repetition.") This is why excess weight sneaks up on us. It's not as if we don't notice it, but because it comes on gradually and unintentionally, it gains a toehold.

Making yourself more aware of the habits that caused you to put on pounds in the first place is a giant step on your journey to optimal weight. The second, more important step is to replace these habits with a healthy lifestyle that over time will become second nature. Until these new habits are locked in and you're well on your way toward your target weight, this is going to require conscientious effort and attention.

Setting goals, scheduling exercise, and deciding on specific refinements in your diet—and then establishing a baseline and periodically recording your progress—will start you off with a strong foundation. Taking the time to write these things down keeps them in the forefront of your mind and has been scientifically demonstrated to provide motivation and improve compliance. Let's begin with everyone's favorite focus and, in many cases, obsession: weight.

REGULAR SELF-WEIGHING HELPS WITH WEIGHT CONTROL

Some people can't walk by a scale without stepping on it, while others don't even own one. What is the better approach for weight loss and maintenance? Most experts agree that regular weigh-ins are associated with better control and a reduced risk of obesity.[1]

In a 2011 study published in the *International Journal of Behavioral Medicine*, Jeffrey VanWormer and colleagues compared the frequency of self-weighing with weight fluctuations over 2 years in a group of 1,222 adults who were part of a larger clinical trial. Not surprisingly, they found that people who were obese initially were more likely to weigh themselves often, and those who did so daily had a 9.7 pound average weight loss during that period. Among the normal-weight individuals, who were the least likely to step on the scale, self-weighing just once a month was linked with a 2.4 pound weight gain.[2]

There's some controversy as to how often you should weigh yourself. Weight Watchers recommends once a week, while others promote daily or monthly self-weighing. I'm sure you know that weight fluctuates from day to day and hour to hour, depending on when and what you eat and drink, your exercise intensity, when you go to the bathroom, and, for women, where you are in your menstrual cycle. Some maintain that daily weighing can be discouraging and depressing because you're more likely to observe normal rises and falls. You could, for example, gain a pound from one day to the next, even if you're doing everything right. My advice is to do what works for you. Although the bulk of the research favors the more frequent approach, if you prefer to weigh yourself once a week or twice a month, go for it. Everyone agrees, however, that weigh-ins should be done at the same time every day, ideally first thing in the morning before exercising and eating.

Another piece of advice, especially in the early stages of your mini-fast with exercise program, is to avoid fixating on the numbers on your scale. Because you are exercising, you are gaining muscle mass at the same time that you're losing fat. This may not show up right away as pounds lost on the scale. In fact, your loss in body fat will likely be more significant than your weight loss at first. So in the first 2 or 3 weeks, your rate of weight loss may not be all that impressive.

Furthermore, digital scales give readouts to the tenth of a pound, and, if yours is like mine, often register slightly different weights if you step on and off it several times in succession. This makes it easy to obsess over minor and insignificant variations. Don't be discouraged if the pounds aren't falling off. Rest assured that your body composition (ratio of fat to muscle) is getting better, your waist is shrinking, and your overall health is improving. After about a month on the program, the pounds will catch up.

THE INFAMOUS PLATEAU

What if you started out with a roar but now seem to be in a holding pattern? This common and extremely frustrating scenario can occur on any weight loss program. You are chugging along, exercising most mornings, fasting until noon every day, eating pretty well, and feeling highly motivated because you're losing a pound or two a week. Then, after several weeks, the weight loss stops in its tracks. You keep it up, but your much-anticipated weekly step onto the scale reveals no change. You try it again, and the readout barely budges. Another week passes, and you experience the same thing.

You may be trading muscle for fat—as I've said, the scale isn't gospel. You may also be minimizing the impact of smaller amounts of weight loss. Half a pound a week doesn't sound like much, but it adds up to 26 pounds over the course of a year, which isn't too shabby.

You may also be experiencing the infamous plateau. Here's why. In Chapter 4, I told you about basal metabolic rate (BMR). This is the energy your body requires for respiration, digestion, circulation, and other vital functions that are active even when you are resting. Your BMR is dependent on a number of factors, and one of them is body mass. Therefore, contrary to popular belief, heavy people have higher BMRs than thin people. When you lose weight, your BMR actually goes down a bit, and you burn fewer calories to maintain these basic physiological operations. Plateauing simply means that you've hit a new equilibrium with your current exercise level and caloric intake. This is less likely to happen on the Mini-Fast Diet because, unlike many weight loss programs, you are exercising and building muscle. Nevertheless, to get things going again, either be more careful about what you eat, increase your activity, or try the optional supplements.

WAIST-TO-HIP RATIO: AN EXCELLENT MARKER OF WEIGHT AND HEALTH

In addition to weighing yourself, I encourage you to use other measuring and tracking techniques, and one of the most reliable is waist-to-hip ratio. A large waist is a clear sign of unhealthy weight—but it's also the most responsive to weight loss efforts such as the mini-fast with exercise.

You may not like the look of fat on your hips, thighs, or legs, but it presents a far less significant health risk. The type of fat in this pear-shape distribution, which is much more common in females than in males, is subcutaneous, meaning that it's stored under the skin. It is the stuff you can grab with your hands and the cellulite that is the bane of many women, including those who are slender. Large hips, provided they're accompanied by a relatively small waist, are actually protective against cardiovascular disease.[3]

Belly fat may also be subcutaneous. Love handles, which are soft and jiggly and can be pinched between your fingers, are subcutaneous, and excessive amounts in this area may also pose a health hazard. However, the most dangerous type, and unfortunately the most common, is intra-abdominal fat, or visceral adipose tissue. If you have a big belly that's firm and hard, rather than squishy and mushy, I hate to disillusion you, but it's visceral fat rather than muscle. This is the fatty tissue that resides deep inside the abdominal cavity, around the liver, colon, kidneys, and other organs. It's the apple-shape obesity associated with metabolic syndrome, cardiovascular disease, type 2 diabetes, and hypertension.

The old view of fat as an inert storehouse has given way to the understanding that visceral adipose tissue is in fact an endocrine organ that plays a role in energy balance, insulin sensitivity, and inflammation.[4] Adipose tissue releases dozens of hormones such as appetite-controlling leptin and insulin-sensitizing adiponectin, along with enzymes, immune modulators, inflammatory chemicals, cytokines, and other substances that have profound effects on tissues throughout the body.

Visceral abdominal fat also floods the system with free fatty acids, which interfere with insulin sensitivity, elevate blood lipids, and damage the arteries. Because this fat mass lies nearby key organs, fatty acids are also deposited in the liver, heart, pancreas, muscles, and other places where fat has no business being. Known as ectopic fat (ectopic means "in an abnormal place or position"), it is linked with organ injury and dysfunction.

I know this is discouraging information for those of you who carry your excess weight in this area. But rather than allowing it to get you down, let it motivate you to take action. The good news is that because visceral fat is so metabolically active, it is the first to be mobilized and burned off.

This is why I suggest that, before embarking on the mini-fast with exercise, you get a tape measure and record your waist circumference. While you're at it, measure your hips too. Although tracking waist girth is good enough on an individual basis, waist-to-hip ratio is a very useful measurement for research purposes because it further defines weight distribution. A woman may have a 30-inch waist, which isn't too bad, but if she is short and small-framed with slim, 34-inch hips, she has abdominal obesity.

How big is too big? Abdominal obesity is defined by the National Heart, Lung, and Blood Institute as a waist circumference greater than 40 inches for men and 35 inches for women.[5] The International Diabetes Federation pegs it at more than 35.5 and 31.5 inches for men and women, respectively.[6] And according to a study published in the *Archives of Internal Medicine* involving more than 100,000 people, waist measurements greater than or equal to 47 inches for men and 43 inches for women double the risk of death, regardless of body mass index and weight. (Although it's hard to imagine how anyone with a waist that large could have a normal weight, apparently some of them did.)[7] Waist-to-hip ratio ranges also vary; see the chart on the next page for average recommendations.

WHAT IS YOUR WAIST-TO-HIP RATIO?

Using a tape measure, held taut but not tight, measure your waist at the narrowest point or, if you have a large waist, 1 inch above the navel. Measure your hips at their broadest point, or around the hip joints. To determine your waist-to-hip ratio, divide the hip into the waist measurement.

Waist-to-Hip Ratio	Men	Women
Ideal:	0.8	0.7
Low Risk	≤ 0.95	≤ 0.8
Moderate Risk	0.96–0.99	0.81–0.84
High Risk:	≥ 1.0	≥ 0.85

So get out your tape measure, record your girth, and start the mini-fast with exercise. Then track your progress, and watch your waist shrink. Because men usually have more visceral fat, they tend to lose weight more rapidly. In 12 weeks, Brian lost 31 pounds and 7½ inches off his waist, and although Raymond dropped only 4 pounds, his waist shrank by 6 inches! But women also respond well. Both Eva and Maria lost 2½ inches and two clothing sizes. This is proof that the mini-fast with exercise turns up your furnace and burns off visceral fat.

BMI: MOST POPULAR, LEAST ACCURATE

The most popular measurement used in regard to weight is body mass index (BMI). Determined by a formula involving weight relative to height, it's utilized to classify people as being underweight, normal weight, overweight, or obese. The best thing BMI has going for it is that it's a single straightforward, easily understood number, which is why it's widely accepted in scientific research, by insurance companies to set premiums, by statisticians to figure obesity rates, and by physicians in clinical practice. The problem is, it isn't accurate.

BMI takes only height and weight into consideration and completely ignores bone density, lean muscle, and fat distribution. Therefore, it overestimates body fat in strong, athletic individuals and underestimates it in older or inactive people. If you have dense bones, a muscular physique, and little body fat, you could easily have a high BMI indicative of obesity. Likewise, if you get no exercise and have little muscle, thinning bones, and a high percentage of body fat, you may have a normal or a low BMI. Who really has the better body composition: the "obese" athlete, the "normal" couch potato, or the frail, elderly person? Obese people definitely have elevated BMIs, but that does not necessarily mean that individuals with elevated BMIs are fat. Another weakness of the BMI? The arbitrary demarcations. Case in point: A 6-foot-tall man is considered normal at 183 pounds but overweight at 184—it's illogical.

Many scientists believe that waist-to-hip ratio, because it takes into account the all-important fat distribution rather than simply weight, is the most reliable and accurate predictor of obesity and health status. Researchers from David Geffen School of Medicine at the University of California, Los Angeles, have found that it's also a dependable forecaster of premature death. Using data from the MacArthur Successful Aging Study, a clinical trial of high-functioning older men and women, they compared all-cause mortality over a 12-year period with BMI, waist circumference, and waist-to-hip circumference ratio. They found clear and direct relationships between waist-to-hip ratio and risk of death. BMI? No association at all.[8]

At my clinic, we do not use BMI to assess our patients' fitness and health. We rely instead on more meaningful markers, such as waist and hip measurements and body composition analysis. But because BMI is commonly used in research and therefore is referred to occasionally in this book, you may use the chart below to figure out your BMI. However, if your doctor bugs you about your BMI, speak up and ask for more sophisticated testing. And don't necessarily believe you're fat just because your BMI says you are.

BODY COMPOSITION ANALYSIS

The human body is composed of 22 organs, 206 bones, more than 600 muscles, and who knows how many trillions of cells. But

BMI

Height	Weight (lbs)													
5'0"	97	102	107	112	118	123	128	133	138	143	148	153	158	163
5'1"	100	106	111	116	122	127	132	137	143	148	153	158	164	169
5'2"	104	109	115	120	126	131	136	142	147	153	158	164	169	175
5'3"	107	113	118	124	130	135	141	146	152	158	163	169	175	180
5'4"	110	116	122	128	134	140	145	151	157	163	169	174	180	186
5'5"	114	120	126	132	138	144	150	156	162	168	174	180	186	192
5'6"	118	124	130	136	142	148	155	161	167	173	179	186	192	198
5'7"	121	127	134	140	146	153	159	166	172	178	185	191	198	204
5'8"	125	131	138	144	151	158	164	171	177	184	190	197	203	210
5'9"	128	135	142	149	155	162	169	176	182	189	196	203	209	216
5'10"	132	139	146	153	160	167	174	181	188	195	202	209	216	222
5'11"	136	143	150	157	165	172	179	186	193	200	208	215	222	229
6'0"	140	147	154	162	169	177	184	191	199	206	213	221	228	235
6'1"	144	151	159	166	174	182	189	197	204	212	219	227	235	242
6'2"	148	155	163	171	179	186	194	202	210	218	225	233	241	249
BMI	19	20	21	22	23	24	25	26	27	28	29	30	31	32

when we talk about body composition, we're talking about the percentages of lean tissue, which includes the muscles, bones, and organs, and adipose tissue, or fat. Accurate body composition analysis is the most precise definer of obesity. A person could have a normal weight, waist-hip measurements, and BMI and still have too much fat. Conversely, though less likely, he could appear to be above normal in all of these parameters but have a decent fat–lean tissue ratio.

Several methods are used to determine body composition. The old-school method, hydrostatic weighing, involves submersion in water. Although it's quite precise and is still used, it has largely been replaced by newer, less cumbersome technologies. Skin calipers estimate the percentage of fat by taking skin-fold measurements, but their accuracy depends upon the skills of the person doing the test, and that can vary considerably.

Bioelectrical impedance analysis (BIA) uses electrical signals to ascertain fat percentage. It works on the premise that because water makes up a significant proportion of muscle and other lean tissues, while fat contains almost no water, electricity travels faster through lean tissue. These devices send a very low-level electrical current through the body and, based on how rapidly it moves, give you an idea of how much body fat and lean tissue you have. BIA is quick, easy, and inexpensive, and we use it at Whitaker Wellness, particularly for patients on a weight loss regimen who return to the clinic weekly or biweekly. A concrete demonstration of fat reduction, even when weight is relatively stable, builds confidence and assures patients that they're on the right track.

The system we use requires the patient to lie down with sensors placed on the hand and the foot, and it is individually calibrated for age, sex, height, build, fitness level, and other variables. Even in a clinical setting, body composition percentages obtained by BIA aren't always correct. For example, it's highly sensitive to hydration; dehydration, which is not uncommon, skews results, in most cases overestimating body fat percentage. That's one reason I'm unconvinced of the accuracy of BIAs on bathroom scales. These increasingly popular features require only that you enter some basic information and step on the scale. Based on an electrical current that travels from foot to foot, these devices determine your fat percentage.

When *Consumer Reports* tested a number of these scales a few years ago, their overall accuracy was rated as "mediocre."[9] If you use such a scale, follow the manufacturer's instructions for programming it, make sure you're hydrated, and use the same guidelines as for weighing (the same time every day, before exercising and eating, etc.). Also, be aware that BIA is sensitive to air and skin temperature as well as to hydration. Most important, take your body fat reading with a grain of salt. One thing these home monitors are useful for, however, is tracking your progress. Even if your fat percentage is not entirely accurate, you may be able to establish a baseline and observe decreases in your body fat as you progress on the Mini-Fast Diet.

Today's gold standard for body composition analysis is dual-energy x-ray absorptiometry (DXA). Done in a medical facility in about 10 minutes, DXA utilizes very low levels of radiation to provide a precise and detailed look at the body's lean and fatty tissues, their specific distribution, and bone mineral density. Because of its exceptional accuracy and high reproducibility, DXA is used more and more often in scientific studies, but it does require special equipment and is relatively expensive.

We use DXA at Whitaker Wellness primarily to measure bone mineral density, so we were fortunate to be able to use it to monitor the before-and-after results of our mini-fast with exercise study participants. Comparisons of before-and-after scans were remarkable—you literally could see the fat disappear.

BODY FAT PERCENTAGES

	WOMEN (% FAT)	MEN (% FAT)
ESSENTIAL FAT	10–12	2–4
ATHLETES	14–20	6–13
FITNESS	21–24	14–17
ACCEPTABLE	25–31	18–25
US AVERAGE[10]	39.9	28.1

I don't think it's necessary for you to rush out and get a body composition analysis. In fact, at the clinic I refrain from ordering this test unless I know that the patient is serious about weight loss. Heavy people already know they're overweight—they don't need a fancy scan to tell them that. However, on a program like the mini-fast with exercise, periodic testing can not only be informative but also, as you watch your fat stores recede, quite empowering. Just make sure it's done with a reliable testing tool.

THE MAN (OR WOMAN) IN THE MIRROR

The easiest and likely the best way to monitor your progress on the mini-fast with exercise is to look in the mirror. Notice how your body contours are changing and see how your clothes fit. Ask yourself how you feel. Do you have more energy? Are your strength and stamina improving? If you have diabetes or hypertension and monitor your blood sugar or blood pressure, are they changing? These considerations matter far more than any formula or calculation.

At the conclusion of the mini-fast clinical trial we conducted at Whitaker Wellness, we interviewed everyone who completed the program. Some lost significant amounts of weight during the

12-week study. Eve lost 17 pounds; Darryl, 18 pounds; Jack, 29 pounds; and Brian, 31 pounds. Equally impressive were Janice's and Sarah's accomplishment: Each lost 4 inches around the waist, which translates into a reduction of two clothing sizes. Meanwhile, Duane lost "only" 10 pounds, but his hemoglobin A1C (a blood test used to monitor patients with diabetes) fell by more than 2 percentage points. And Javier, a young man who was discovered to have diabetes during his initial evaluation for the study, dropped 30 pounds and 7½ inches around his waist, and his blood sugar fell into the normal range—with no treatment other than the mini-fast with exercise and weight loss. We also saw remarkable improvements in cholesterol, triglycerides, and insulin sensitivity.

As you'll see from the photographs and the stories scattered throughout the book, mini-fasters across the board are looking great and feeling energetic, encouraged, and confident that they've found the ticket to weight control and optimal health.

RECORD YOUR JOURNEY

Once you gather all this information, what do you do with it? I recommend that you record it. Taking the time to write it down, even though it may be for your eyes only, is in itself a statement of your seriousness and intention to follow the program.

Begin with baseline data: current weight, waist and hip measurements (and ratio, if you want to do the math), as well as general comments about how you feel, your medical condition, and medication usage. If you check your blood pressure or blood sugar levels, note them, too. And if you have had recent blood tests and know your levels of cholesterol (total, HDL, and LDL), triglycerides, and perhaps C-reactive protein and liver enzymes, be sure to record them. All of these numbers will likely improve with weight loss.

Once you get started on the program, keep a daily log of your exercise sessions and mini-fasts, comments on your diet and overall experience, and your weight, if you're weighing every day. (See the sample tracking sheet on pages 150–151.) You may also want to pay closer attention to your diet and jot down what you eat and when you eat it. Neither this nor calorie counting is a requirement, but some people find that it makes them more aware of what they put in their mouths. Elizabeth, who lost 25 pounds in the 13 months between her engagement and wedding, wrote down every single thing she ate for 6 months. It forced her to be realistic about her food choices and see where improvements could and should be made.

In addition to monitoring your daily activities, review your progress regularly and summarize it week by week. This will give you an at-a-glance picture of how you're doing over the longer term, which is when the real results roll in. One final suggestion: Post your goals, activity logs, and progress notes on your fridge or keep them at your desk, where they will be a frequent reminder of your good intentions.

You are embarking on a very important, potentially life-changing journey. Your success will have far-reaching effects on virtually every aspect of your life: your health, your appearance, your mood and energy, your self-esteem, and perhaps even your relationships with others. Tracking your progress is a powerful tool that will help you stay on the path and arrive at your intended destination.

THE MINI-FAST DIET

Mini-Fast with Exercise Daily Tracking

BASELINE DATA

Date: _____   Waist Circumference: _____

Weight: _____   Hip Circumference: _____

Lab Numbers (if desired): _____

Exercise: Aim for 5 days a week (3 minimum), during the fasting period, of moderately strenuous aerobic exercise, building up to a minimum of 40 minutes per session.

Mini-Fast: No food until lunchtime (or between breakfast and dinner, should you choose that option), drink lots of water and, if desired, noncaloric beverages.

Supplements (optional): Ketosis Essentials: one scoop before exercise, another scoop during the mini-fast to curb appetite (if needed); Metabolic Essentials: two capsules twice a day with meals.

Diet: Calorie counting isn't necessary, but for best results eat a healthy, relatively low-fat diet with low-glycemic carbohydrates and moderate amounts of lean protein.

DAY	DID YOU EXERCISE? (ACTIVITY, TIME, AND DURATION)	DID YOU MINI-FAST?	DID YOU TAKE THE OPTIONAL SUPPLE-MENTS?	HOW WAS YOUR DIET? (GOOD, FAIR, OR POOR)	WEIGHT
SUN.					
MON.					
TUES.					
WED.					
THURS.					
FRI.					
SAT.					

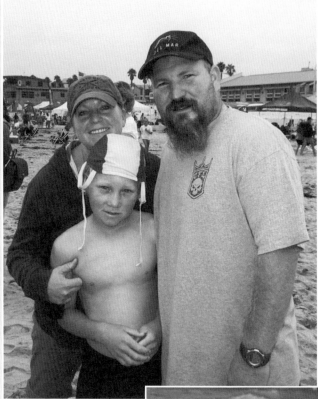

Stephanie and Jack Pacheco prior to starting the program

. . . and after 12 weeks on the mini-fast diet with exercise (above)

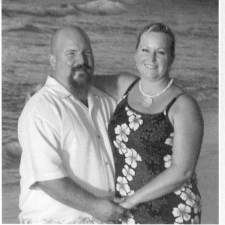

Stephanie and Jack Pacheco: "Find a Partner to Do It With"

Stephanie and Jack Pacheco are a great couple in their late thirties who live in California with their four sons. Jack and Stephanie learned about our mini-fast with exercise study from a friend whose mother works at the clinic, at a time when they were looking for something that would get them motivated to lose weight. A high school football player and college wrestler, Jack was exceptionally active when he was younger. But as the years rolled by and he got busy with family and work, he did less and less—and gained more and more, finally topping out at 233 pounds. Stephanie's weight gain was less extreme, but she too was ready to make some changes.

The Pachecos were perfect study participants because they were very compliant. They both exercised 5 days a week. Stephanie walked or used machines at the gym, and Jack jogged, an activity he used to love but had gotten out of the habit of doing. Now he was back with a vengeance. Skipping breakfast took some getting used to. Stephanie, in particular, felt hungry at first, but it got easier, especially when she took the supplements that are an optional part of the program. Although they ate a regular lunch and dinner and had snacks, they watched their diets. They tried to stay away from sweets and excess carbs; ate a lot of chicken, salads, and vegetables; and enjoyed a number of our suggested recipes.

During those 12 weeks, Jack lost 29 pounds and nearly 5 inches from his waist. Stephanie lost 13 pounds—virtually all of it fat—and 2½ inches. Equally remarkable, we had discovered on their initial blood tests that both Jack and Stephanie had diabetes, and their fasting blood sugar and hemoglobin A1C (which gives a broader picture of longer-term average blood sugar levels) were elevated. After 12 weeks on the Mini-Fast Diet, all of those numbers fell into the normal range.

Stephanie said, "Doing this with my husband made it much easier. We kept each other 'honest' in our daily exercise and our eating habits. If I could give advice to anyone contemplating this program, it would be to find a partner to do it with. For us, it made all the difference in the world."

Susie Heald: Lost 27 Pounds and Kept Them Off

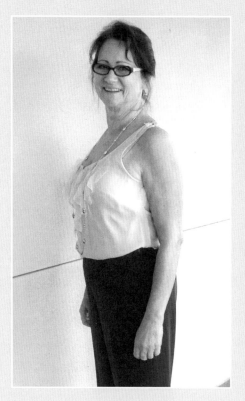

"For most of my life, I was pretty small, and any time I gained weight, I could lose it with little effort. After turning 40, however, I seemed to put on several pounds every year, and I just couldn't take them off. Over the years I tried Lindora and Weight Watchers, which I liked because you can just pick up their frozen foods in the store and don't really have to pay attention to what you're eating. But that didn't work for long—eating packaged food as a steady diet is very unhealthy and boring. When I hit 160 pounds, I signed up for a program that delivered fresh, healthy, low-calorie meals. I did this for 4 months and lost 10 to 12 pounds. I also lost a lot of money, as this food was very expensive. And within 8 months of discontinuing these meals, the weight returned because I hadn't put any effort into learning how to be healthy on my own.

"When I heard about the mini-fast with exercise program, it seemed like something I could do. I'm one of those people who can go all day without eating. I never get hungry until about 11:30 or noon, so it's easy for me to skip breakfast. Evenings are another story. When I get home after work, I used to eat cheese, potato salad, and anything else in sight, and I could practically live on bread and sweets. But once I realized the number of calories in the things I was eating—not to mention how easy it is to eat healthy food that tastes good—it became easier. Now I never eat bread or pasta, and I seldom eat sweets.

"Instead, I eat lots of salads—my husband is really creative with salads and throws in all kinds of tasty things like chicken, fish, vegetables, and fruit. I also eat much smaller portions. At home we use smaller plates, which make a huge difference. When we go out, my husband and I share a meal. (It is amazing the amount of food you get in restaurants!) And we never eat the bread they serve before dinner. I am not saying we're perfect, but when we cheat, it is usually with popcorn.

"Exercising in the mornings was easy at first because I was excited about this new approach, but it's difficult to stay motivated. You have to find the right exercise for you. For me, it's walking for 30 minutes and—since I love to dance—Jazzercise, which I do three times a week. It is so much fun, you don't even know you're working out. In addition, I enjoy yoga on my Wii because it's good to stretch and it's easy on the body. I also take the recommended supplements. Sometimes it's hard to remember to take them every day, but you don't realize how good they make you feel until you stop taking them.

"My initial goal when I started the mini-fast was 148 pounds. I have achieved that and more. I now weigh 133, and my pants size has gone from a 12 to a 10 and sometimes an 8, depending on the brand.

"My advice to anyone who is considering this program is to just do it. I like to think of the overnight fast as dieting while you're sleeping. What could be easier? If you love breakfast food, just eat it for lunch. You do have to pay attention to what you eat, but you will soon find that you can live without all the useless, unhealthy foods out there. Plus, you'll discover that there are tons of really tasty, healthy things to eat.

"Finally, you have to stay motivated. Just putting on clothes that aren't tight is a great motivator for me, and having friends and family comment on how I look doesn't hurt. My husband and I also weigh ourselves every day on our Wii, which tracks weight and BMI. If I gain more than 2 pounds, I get more serious about the program until I get back to my ideal weight. When you know your husband is weighing with you every morning, you want to stay on track. Besides, we are a little competitive!"

CHAPTER 8

REMOVING YOUR ROADBLOCKS

My weight kept creeping up, and it bothered me terribly. I had always been energetic and weight-conscious, and I was an avid exerciser until constant fatigue slowed me down. After I got on natural thyroid, I started to feel like a normal person, like the person I used to be. I began walking again and paying attention to my diet, and I am happy to report that I've lost 21 pounds and know that I will lose more.

—JOYCE

If you've had trouble losing weight in the past, despite sincere and conscientious efforts to reduce calories and exercise regularly, an underlying medical problem may be part of your problem. It's important that you look for and correct such conditions. Otherwise, even if you go full-bore on the mini-fast with exercise program, you'll have one foot on the gas pedal and the other on the brake.

A handful of well-recognized disorders can cause weight gain. I had a patient, Charmaine, who came to me with congestive heart failure, which occurs when the weakened heart muscle is unable to pump with enough force and fluids accumulate in the lungs and lower limbs. Wheelchair-bound, she struggled to breathe, and her legs were so swollen with edema that the skin had split. I started her on high doses of coenzyme Q10, L-carnitine, and other nutritional supplements to enhance her heart function. Within 8 weeks she had lost 64 pounds—all of it excess fluid—her lungs cleared, and her heart returned to normal.

Kidney and liver failure can also result in fluid retention and weight gain; and Cushing's syndrome, caused by an excess of cortisol, is marked by an accumulation of fat in the face, back, and abdomen. These are serious diseases accompanied by other signs and symptoms that all physicians know to look for. However, more subtle conditions that contribute to obesity and thwart weight loss are often overlooked. The comprehensive evaluation that patients undergo at the Whitaker Wellness Institute includes ruling out *all* undiagnosed issues that may be packing on pounds and short-circuiting weight loss efforts. We begin by testing hormone levels.

COULD IT BE YOUR THYROID?

The thyroid gland produces hormones that are the primary regulator of your body's basal metabolic rate—the energy you expend when you are completely at rest—as well as overall energy expenditure.[1] Therefore, it's not surprising that thyroid dysfunction could influence weight, and that hypothyroidism, or low thyroid function, is often associated with weight gain.

Hypothyroidism is far more common than you might expect. It affects up to 10 percent of all Americans and as many as one in five women over age 65. Unfortunately, about half of those suffering with this condition are unaware that their thyroid could be contributing to their fatigue, depression, chronic constipation, dry skin, thinning hair, cold hands and feet, elevated cholesterol and triglycerides, and/or weight issues. After all, these problems could easily be blamed on any number of other conditions. Conventional physicians frequently overlook thyroid dysfunction as a potential link and, far too often, simply write these symptoms off as inevitable aspects of aging.

At best, they may run blood tests to evaluate thyroid function. The usual "rule out" test is thyroid-stimulating hormone (TSH). TSH is produced in the pituitary gland and acts like an on/off switch for thyroid hormone synthesis. When the pituitary senses that blood levels of thyroid hormones are low, it secretes TSH, which signals the thyroid gland to release more hormones. Therefore, a high TSH level on a blood test is an indication of hypothyroidism. Most doctors let it go at that. If your TSH level is within the normal range, low thyroid is ruled out, end of story.

This is not the best approach. The TSH test is far from foolproof, and patients with a normal TSH level may nevertheless have insufficient levels of active thyroid hormones. In a study conducted in Israel, researchers enrolled women who had either hypothyroidism or subclinical hypothyroidism (blood tests in the upper range of normal—which few physicians would treat). The researchers measured the women's blood pressure, body mass index (BMI), cognitive status, triglycerides, LDL, HDL, and total cholesterol levels, then started them on thyroid replacement therapy. After 3 months on supplemental thyroid, the participants were retested, and there were improvements across the board. Blood pressures were lower, lipid profiles and cognitive function improved, and average weight and BMI went down.[2]

At Whitaker Wellness, we treat patients, not lab tests. If all the signs and symptoms of hypothyroidism are present, even if the TSH level is near normal, we often give patients a trial of natural thyroid replacement to see if it makes a difference. And it often does. One of my patients, Stephanie, is a woman in her early thirties who is a real go-getter—hard working, high achieving, and always going in 10 directions at once. That's why she was so distressed when she began feeling tired, sluggish, and lethargic. In addition, despite regular workouts and no changes in her diet, she was gaining weight. Although her TSH and other markers of thyroid function all came back normal, I prescribed a trial of low-dose natural thyroid and requested that she monitor her basal body temperature (see "How to Test Your Basal Body Temperature" on page 160). Over the next few months, her temperatures rose from the low 96s—an indication of hypothyroidism—into the normal range, her energy bounced back, and her weight loss efforts got back on track.

Synthroid versus Natural Thyroid

The most popular thyroid replacement drug is Synthroid (levothyroxine). Synthroid is a synthetic version of one thyroid hormone, T4 (thyroxine). I've never understood conventional medicine's infatuation with this drug. Although T4 is the most abundant thyroid hormone, it must be converted in the body into T3 (triiodothyronine), which is the more active form. Some people, particularly as they get older, do not efficiently convert T4 into T3, which may explain both the age-related rise in hypothyroidism and why Synthroid fails to work in some patients.

At Whitaker Wellness, we prescribe natural thyroid replacement, such as Armour or Naturethroid. Derived from natural

HOW TO TEST YOUR BASAL BODY TEMPERATURE

Because thyroid hormones regulate your basal body metabolism—the energy you expend at rest—testing your basal body temperature can give you a ballpark indication of your thyroid function. I want to make it clear that this test is not infallible nor is it the be-all and end-all in thyroid diagnostics. However, it is something you can do on your own at home to glean another piece of information on your journey toward optimal weight.

✔ Get a glass mercury thermometer (the old-fashioned kind) or a basal body temperature thermometer at a drugstore.

✔ Before going to sleep at night, shake it down and place it on your nightstand or within reach.

✔ First thing in the morning—while still in bed and with as little movement as possible—place the sensor end of the thermometer in your armpit and tuck your arm against your side to hold it in place. Lie motionless for exactly 10 minutes. Record the temperature.

✔ Repeat this for three consecutive mornings and average your temperature readings.

✔ Women who are menstruating should test on the third, fourth, and fifth days of their cycles. Everyone else can test at any time.

✔ Normal readings are between 97.8 and 98.2 degrees Fahrenheit. Temperatures consistently lower than 97.6 degrees are suggestive of hypothyroidism.

✔ Discuss your findings with your physician, and, if appropriate, ask for a clinical trial of natural thyroid.

desiccated porcine thyroid, these products contain T3, T4, as well as T1, T2, and the entire gamut of thyroid hormones. Patients who had been on synthetic thyroid drugs often blossom after switching to natural thyroid. Alice took Synthroid for decades but was unable to lose weight or clear up a host of health problems. Within 8 months of switching to Armour natural thyroid, she lost 30 pounds, had energy to burn, and reported improvements in her overall health.

For general thyroid support, make sure that you're getting enough selenium and iodine. Studies show that 200 micrograms per day of selenium reduces the risk of—and is an excellent adjunct treatment for—Hashimoto's thyroiditis, an autoimmune disorder and a common cause of hypothyroidism.[3] Iodine is required for the synthesis of thyroid hormones, and deficiencies in this mineral are widespread. Average levels today are just half of what they were 30 years ago, thanks to poor diet and environmental factors that interfere with iodine uptake, such as fluoride in water, thiocyanate in cigarette smoke, and perchlorate, a contaminant from rocket fuel that is pervasive in our water and food.[4] Your best bet is to take a good daily multivitamin that contains 150 micrograms of iodine and 200 micrograms of selenium.

Do not underestimate the importance of robust thyroid function. In addition to weight gain and other symptoms noted above, hypothyroidism also increases the risk of heart attack, immune dysfunction, and infertility. Furthermore, because these hormones play an integral role in fetal growth and brain development, women's poor thyroid function during pregnancy may be related to their children's risk of neurological problems.[5]

SEX HORMONES AND WEIGHT

Other hormones are also associated with weight gain. Estrogen, the primary female sex hormone, promotes fat storage, particularly in the hips and thighs, which explains why women have a considerably greater percentage of fat versus lean body mass than men. It's all about reproduction—adequate fat is necessary for successful pregnancy and fetal development. Fat is so important for pregnancy that, when body fat drops too low, as it sometimes does in serious athletes, professional dancers, and people with anorexia,

BIOIDENTICAL HORMONES: SAFE AND EFFECTIVE

Many women are uncomfortable with the idea of hormone replacement therapy, and with good reason. Several years ago, the Women's Health Initiative (WHI), a large, government-funded clinical trial that evaluated Prempro (a combination of Premarin, a conjugated estrogen drug made from horse urine, and Provera, a synthetic progestin), was terminated early when it was discovered that women taking this drug had an increased risk of breast cancer, stroke, blood clots, and heart attacks. Although subsequent reviews of the WHI data have minimized some of these dangers, as far as I'm concerned, no woman should ever use these drugs—especially since safe, natural alternatives are readily available.

Bioidentical hormones are identical to those produced in the human body. Because these are compounds that the body is intimately familiar with, most of the concerns that arise with conventional hormones are null and void. A 2009 review of published studies concluded, "Physiological data and clinical outcomes demonstrate that bioidentical hormones are associated with lower risks, including the risk of breast cancer and cardiovascular disease, and are more efficacious than their synthetic and animal-derived counterparts. Until evidence is found to the contrary, bioidentical hormones remain the preferred method of HRT [hormone replacement therapy]."[6]

menstruation stops. Women may gripe about big hips and thighs, but as we discussed in the previous chapter, this fat distribution is much healthier than abdominal fat.

Then menopause hits. Many of my female patients swear up and down that "The Change" exacerbated their weight problems. Furthermore, they tell me that even if they aren't gaining much, their fat is migrating to their bellies. Men and women alike tend to lose muscle mass and gain fat as they get older and

Natural hormones are also better tolerated, particularly if they're formulated by a compounding pharmacy. The usual hormone replacement drugs come in standardized dosages and delivery systems—one or two sizes fit all—another reason so many women have a hard time adjusting to conventional hormones. Bioidentical hormones, however, may be prescribed in a wide range of doses and combinations tailored for each patient. For example, if a woman is dealing with a low libido, her doctor may request that a little testosterone be added to her estrogen cream (testosterone is the hormone of desire in both sexes). Or if dryness is an issue, special vaginal preparations can be made. These prescriptions are sent to a compounding pharmacist, who prepares them individually per the doctor's orders.

Although bioidentical hormones are making inroads, many physicians still opt for the conventional drugs. If your doctor won't work with you on this, it's worth the effort to find one who will. Using bioidentical hormone replacement therapy to restore your hormone levels to those of a young woman can make a world of difference in how you feel and look. To locate a compounding pharmacy that formulates bioidentical hormones and can refer you to a prescribing physician, call the International Academy of Compounding Pharmacists (IACP) at 800-927-4227 or go to iacprx.org.

become less active. But hormones are also involved. Declining levels of estrogen and progesterone, accompanied by a relative increase in androgens (male hormones), clearly play a role in the shift toward abdominal fat accumulation experienced by many postmenopausal women. And some experts believe that as estrogen production in the ovaries peters out and ovulation ceases, fat cells, which also produce this hormone, pick up the slack and become overactive.

I'm a wholehearted supporter of bioidentical hormone replacement therapy for women who are in this stage of life. Bioidentical estrogen, balanced with natural progesterone—hormones that are exactly like those produced by the human body—relieve hot flashes, night sweats, poor sleep, irritability, mood swings, and difficulty concentrating. They restore energy and a sense of well-being, and make exercise and other positive lifestyle activities more achievable. I am aware that a number of women contend that hormone replacement makes them gain weight, but there is no scientific support for this. Conventional hormones, particularly synthetic progesterone wannabes such as Provera, may cause fluid retention in some women, but bioidentical hormones are more likely to promote weight loss rather than weight gain.

Most women who use bioidentical hormone replacement therapy love it. Some of you may recall Oprah Winfrey's experience, which she shared publicly a few years ago. Feeling tired, run-down, and out of balance and having difficulty sleeping and regulating her weight, she finally took the advice of a friend and visited a doctor well versed in bioidentical hormones. He reviewed her lab work and started her on a hormone regimen. "After 1 day on bioidentical estrogen," Oprah said, "I felt the veil lift. After 3 days, the sky was bluer; my brain was no longer fuzzy; my memory was sharper. I was literally singing and had a skip in my step."

My patients may not feel as poetically inspired as Oprah was, but we consistently get excellent feedback. Bioidentical hormones must be prescribed by a physician and can be made to order by a compounding pharmacist.

TESTOSTERONE, BIG BELLIES, AND MAN BOOBS

Men are also affected by fluctuating hormone levels. In their early to mid-thirties, guys who were able to eat whatever they wanted and not worry about gaining an ounce often develop a beer belly or a spare tire that just gets bigger over time. Although much of this has to do with diet and activity level, we can blame some of it on changes in testosterone. Testosterone is the quintessential male hormone—it makes men muscular, hairy, and horny. As we get older, levels of free testosterone, the active form of this hormone, decline. In addition to age-related decreases in hormonal output by the testes, more and more testosterone is bound to proteins and rendered biologically inactive. This fall in free testosterone predisposes men to heart disease, depression, and—you guessed it—changes in body composition, particularly the loss of lean muscle mass.

Another age-related phenomenon is that greater amounts of testosterone are converted into estrogen, and increases in estrogen encourage the deposition of fat. Much of this conversion, which is mediated by an enzyme called aromatase, actually occurs in the adipose, or fat, tissue. The fatter you are, particularly in the abdominal area, the less favorable the testosterone-estrogen balance—and the less favorable this balance, the more likely you are to gain weight. Increases in estrogen also stimulate the growth of breast tissue in men, resulting in a somewhat embarrassing condition that affects a significant percentage of older men called gynecomastia, or "man boobs." (Some medications, which we'll discuss later in this chapter, are also linked with gynecomastia.)

Although many physicians are loath to prescribe testosterone to their male patients, I consider testosterone replacement to be an invaluable therapy. Physiological doses—to restore levels to those of a healthy young man—boost sex drive and performance, increase muscle mass and bone density, and perk up energy and mood. A low testosterone level is a risk factor for type 2 diabetes, cardiovascular disease, and metabolic syndrome, but testosterone replacement reduces the risk. In a 2011 study, Italian researchers looked at the effects of testosterone on metabolic syndrome and concluded that "androgen [testosterone] deprivation increases abdominal adiposity" and testosterone replacement both decreases belly fat and improves insulin sensitivity.[7]

Testosterone requires a prescription, and care must be taken to suppress its conversion to estrogen, but it is an excellent therapy for many age-related problems. In the doses I'm recommending there's no danger of "roid rage" (excessive aggression) or testicular atrophy, which may occur in athletes and bodybuilders who overdo it in an attempt to put on muscle. And although supplemental testosterone should not be used by men who have prostate cancer, as it could fuel malignant cell growth, it does not—I repeat, it does not—*cause* prostate cancer.

CHRONIC STRESS AND WEIGHT GAIN

The adrenal glands, which sit on top of the kidneys, produce a number of hormones, and chief among them are epinephrine (also known as adrenaline) and cortisol, commonly called stress hormones. Whenever you feel threatened or endangered, these hormones kick the fight-or-flight response into high gear, an evolutionary adaptation that increases your heart rate and blood pressure, makes you mentally alert, and provides energy to prepare you for action. To fuel this anticipated burst of energy, cortisol raises blood sugar levels by signaling a process called gluconeogenesis, in which amino acids and other substrates are converted into glucose. Once the perceived danger passes, secretion of these hormones ebbs, and the blood levels of all these substances return to normal.

However, when we're chronically stressed, worried, or fearful, stress hormone levels remain high. Never mind that the perceived threat requires no physical reaction, or that it may even be "all in your head." These hormones make us tense, edgy, and ready to rumble. Another result of a continuously high cortisol level is that it keeps glucose, and thus insulin levels, constantly elevated. And elevated insulin, as you know, shuts down fat burning. It also sets the stage for insulin resistance and, along with it, metabolic syndrome, as well as the accumulation of visceral abdominal fat. This is one of the links between chronic stress and weight gain.

DHEA Blunts the Effects of Chronic Stress

DHEA (dehydroepiandrosterone) is another hormone produced in the adrenal glands. Sometimes called the mother hormone because it is a precursor to testosterone, estrogen, and other sex hormones, DHEA also helps counter the adverse effects of stress. There is an inverse relationship between levels of cortisol and DHEA: The higher the cortisol, the lower the DHEA, and vice versa. Individuals with an elevated cortisol-DHEA ratio often have insulin resistance and excess weight, primarily in the abdominal region. Furthermore, they typically find it next to impossible to shed pounds, despite following a spartan diet and exercising regularly.

By blunting some of the adverse effects of cortisol, DHEA may help prevent and reverse abdominal obesity. When older, overweight men and women with low blood levels of DHEA took 50 milligrams of DHEA daily for 6 months, the men lost 10.2 percent of their visceral adipose tissue and the women lost 7.4 percent. Their insulin sensitivity improved as well.[8] Other studies have shown that DHEA increases bone density, enhances libido and sexual function, and improves mood and sense of well-being. DHEA levels decline with age—an average 25-year-old's is five times higher than that of a 70-year-old. However, chronic stress and a number of disease states are also associated with reduced

SAFFRON AND 5-HTP FOR STRESS EATING

If you are battling food cravings, particularly for high-carbohydrate foods, there are two nutritional supplements you should try: 5-hydroxytryptophan (5-HTP) and saffron. Both of these natural products, available over the counter, curb appetite by increasing levels of serotonin. Although this neurotransmitter is best known for its effects on mood, it also influences hunger and sense of satiety, and low levels may cause uncontrollable appetite, especially for carbohydrates. Dieting can actually make matters worse. Serotonin levels tend to decline in individuals eating low-calorie diets, which may not provide enough of the amino acids necessary for serotonin production in the brain.

5-HTP is the direct precursor to serotonin. When taken in supplement form, it gently but predictably boosts serotonin levels, which improves mood in people suffering with depression, reduces appetite, and tones down carbohydrate cravings.[9] Saffron, derived from crocus flowers *(Crocus sativus)* and used as a culinary spice and as a traditional remedy for digestive problems and inflammation, has also been shown to increase serotonin concentrations. Recent research has shown that saffron extracts not only improve anxiety, mood, and energy[10] but also reduce appetite and between-meals snacking.[11]

levels. Your goal, regardless of your age, should be to bring your DHEA level into the range of a healthy young adult.

Ask your doctor for a blood test of DHEA-sulfate (a DHEA metabolite in the blood). If it falls below the young-adult range, consider taking supplemental DHEA. The usual starting doses are 25 milligrams a day for women and 50 milligrams for men. Retest in 3 or 4 months, and adjust your dose accordingly. DHEA is sold over the counter and does not require a prescription. It is safe and well tolerated. Because DHEA is converted into testosterone in women (that's why it improves energy and libido), too

In a 2010 study, mildly overweight women ages 25 to 45 were randomly divided into two groups. The women in the first group took a 90-milligram capsule of Satiereal, a standardized saffron extract, with breakfast, and another with dinner, while those in the other group were given placebo capsules. For 8 weeks, they were asked to make no diet changes but were required to record all "snacking events" (food eaten outside of mealtime). By the end of the study, there was a 55 percent average reduction in snacking events in the saffron group compared with a 25 percent reduction in the placebo group. Furthermore, the women taking the saffron supplements lost a modest but statistically significant amount of weight (an average of 2.1 pounds), while those taking the placebo had a slight weight gain.[12]

Saffron and 5-HTP are not quick fixes, and you can't expect to take these supplements, sit back, and watch the pounds melt off. However, if stress eating is sabotaging your attempts to control your weight, I suggest trying one of these serotonin enhancers as an adjunct to the mini-fast with exercise. The recommended dose of saffron is 90 milligrams twice a day. For 5-HTP, start with 50 milligrams twice a day, 20 minutes before meals. If you still feel cravings after 4 weeks, you may increase the dosage to 100 milligrams two or three times a day. I do not recommend exceeding this amount.

much may cause oily skin and slight facial hair growth. Cutting back on the dose will rapidly reverse these conditions. DHEA is not recommended for men with prostate cancer or women with breast, ovarian, or endometrial cancer.

Stress and Emotional Eating

Chronic stress is also linked with feelings of disquiet and dissatisfaction, worry and anxiety, fidgeting and restlessness, unhappiness and depression. A popular coping mechanism is eating. People who "stress eat" don't necessarily overeat at mealtime. Rather, they snack throughout the day and into the evening, and the things they eat tend to be high-sugar, high-fat comfort foods that reinforce more snacking.[13] For some, it's the creamy mouthfeel, like ice cream or macaroni and cheese. Others go for sweets—chocolate cravings are a cliché—or salty items such as chips. I have a friend who tells me that, if she doesn't watch herself, she can easily plow through a large bag of potato chips in one sitting.

Galen, whose story you'll read at the end of this chapter, was ruled by emotional eating most of her life. She bounced from one diet to another, losing weight but always gaining it back. It took years—decades, actually—until she got to the point where food no longer had power over her, and she is finally in control of her weight. Emotional eating can undermine the sincerest of weight loss plans, so do what you can to get to the bottom of it.[14] For Galen, it involved the resolution of personal issues and a commitment to exercise, aided and abetted by the mini-fast with exercise. For others, it may require counseling or making significant life changes. It is beyond the scope of this book to offer suggestions for this multifaceted problem. However, it is well worth the effort to understand and solve these issues, not only for your weight but for virtually every aspect of your life.

INSULIN RESISTANCE AND METABOLIC SYNDROME

We discussed insulin resistance and metabolic syndrome as consequences of excess weight in Chapter 2, but I want to briefly revisit these conditions because they are a cause, as well as a result, of obesity. You may not think of insulin as a hormone, but as anyone with type 1 diabetes can tell you, it is one of the body's most important hormones, because without it, nutrients cannot be transported into the cells. Your digestive system breaks down the food you eat into glucose, amino acids, fatty acids, and other basic components. As glucose is released into the blood, the pancreas secretes insulin, which signals the cells to take up glucose and other nutrients.

Sometimes, however, the cells fail to respond to these signals, and more and more insulin must be produced in order to clear glucose out of the blood. This is known as insulin resistance, and it's associated with so many metabolic abnormalities that the cluster of conditions linked to it is called metabolic syndrome. Insulin resistance is both caused by and contributes to weight gain, particularly in the abdominal area. As a matter of fact, the most visible sign of insulin resistance and metabolic syndrome is abdominal obesity.

But the problems are more than skin-deep. As adipocytes (fat cells) in this area balloon with fat, they release fatty acids that drive up levels of triglycerides (fats in the blood). Metabolic syndrome is also accompanied by reduced levels of protective HDL cholesterol; increased concentrations of small, dense LDL; and hypertension—all of which are risk factors for cardiovascular disease. Furthermore, surplus fat has to get deposited elsewhere, and much of it ends up in places where fat has no business being, such as the liver, muscles, and pancreas. This inappropriate deposition, called ectopic fat, leads to chronic inflammation, oxidative stress, additional weight gain, and more severe insulin resistance. To compensate, the pancreas must churn out more and more insulin. Over time, stressed by increased demands and damaged by ectopic fat, it cannot keep up. At that point, type 2 diabetes develops.[15]

Now you can see how tangled and destructive the web of abdominal obesity and insulin resistance can be. It isn't always clear which came first—excess fat or metabolic syndrome—but the endgame is the same: an increased risk of heart disease, diabetes, and premature death. There are natural treatments for insulin resistance and the various aspects of metabolic syndrome, and getting a handle on them may help with your weight loss efforts. (To learn more, visit www.whitakerwellness.com.) However, the most effective treatment for metabolic syndrome is diet and exercise, i.e., the mini-fast with exercise.

H.N. had metabolic syndrome for at least 20 years (low HDL, elevated triglycerides, slightly higher than normal LDL, and a large waist). His doctor put him on Zocor, a cholesterol-lowering drug, but he found the side effects intolerable. So he discontinued it and started taking niacin and following the mini-fast with exercise. In less than 3 months, he lost 17 pounds, his triglycerides decreased and his HDL cholesterol improved, and he was thrilled to have found a way to manage his metabolic syndrome.

Robert Geiger of Port St. Lucie, Florida, has a long history of diabetes and has been on insulin as well as oral medications for

SOS FOR PCOS

Women, if your weight problems are accompanied by irregular periods, acne, and excess body hair, you may have polycystic ovary syndrome (PCOS). Affecting up to 1 in 10 women of childbearing age, PCOS is caused by a storm of hormonal imbalances that include an excess of estrogen, testosterone, and insulin. Although it has the greatest impact on the reproductive organs—the ovaries are swollen with numerous small cysts that may cause infertility—PCOS also has much in common with insulin resistance and metabolic syndrome, including abdominal obesity, lipid abnormalities, hypertension, and an increased risk of heart disease and diabetes. If you suspect that it may be the culprit behind your weight gain, talk to your doctor at once. Therapies typically used to treat type 2 diabetes, promote weight loss, increase insulin sensitivity, and curb testosterone production result in broad improvements for many women with this condition.

DRAMATIC DROP IN BLOOD SUGAR

Beverley H., who followed the mini-fast with exercise protocol as part of the Diabesity Challenge, lost only 4 pounds during the 12-week contest period. Yet her fasting blood sugar improved dramatically, from 356 to 200, and she shed 2 inches from her waist and 4 inches from her hips.

10 years. He also has hypertension and high cholesterol and triglycerides. Robert's response to the mini-fast with exercise was remarkable: "I did not do anything except move breakfast to 12:00 noon. I lost 10 pounds, 2 inches off my hips and waist, and my cholesterol improved a lot."

"A lot" is an understatement. Robert sent in his before-and-after lab reports. His total cholesterol before starting the mini-fast with exercise was 221, and his level of protective HDL cholesterol was low at 42, for a total cholesterol/HDL ratio (a marker of cardiovascular risk) of 5.26, which is in the "red zone." His triglycerides were also high at 287 (normal is less than 150). After 12 weeks on the program, his cholesterol fell to 122—99 points! As if that weren't impressive enough, his HDL level actually increased to 46, bringing his risk ratio down to a very respectable 2.65. His triglycerides also fell into the normal range, and his fasting blood sugar improved as well. Wow! Not surprisingly, Robert was a winner in the *Health & Healing* Diabesity Challenge.

Carl P., from Harrisburg, North Carolina, was another Diabesity Challenge winner. Over the course of 12 weeks, he lost nearly 26 pounds, plus 3 inches from his waist and almost that much from his hips. Carl, who has diabetes and heart disease, also had some pretty dramatic improvements in his blood work. His total,

HDL, and LDL cholesterol went from 246, 57, and 172, respectively, to 166, 78, and 80. This means his total cholesterol/HDL ratio declined from 4.3 to 2.1.

Increasing protective HDL cholesterol is notoriously difficult. Yet on the mini-fast with exercise, Carl's jumped by 21 points!

PRESCRIPTION DRUGS CAN PACK ON THE POUNDS

Iatrogenic means "induced inadvertently in a patient by a physician's activity, manner, or therapy."[16] When a patient dies from a heart attack or stroke while undergoing an angioplasty or bypass surgery, it's considered an iatrogenic death. Say a doctor prescribes a pain-relieving drug that causes an ulcer; that's an iatrogenic injury or disease. Dozens of commonly prescribed medications cause iatrogenic weight gain.[17] That's right—the drugs you're taking could be making you fat.

I see the fallout from iatrogenic weight gain at my clinic every day, particularly in patients with diabetes. Let me give you an example. A patient of mine we'll call Bill had type 2 diabetes for 10 years before coming to the clinic. His physician back home started him on an oral sulfonylurea, a medication in a class of drugs that stimulate insulin production and are notorious for causing weight gain. It worked for a time, but slowly and surely his blood sugar—and his weight—began to rise. So his doctor increased his dosage. Again, Bill's levels improved for a time, but after a while both his blood sugar and the size of his waistline started to creep up. Eventually, the oral drugs stopped working, so his doctor switched him to a low dose of insulin. Over the next few years, his insulin dose was periodically ratcheted up to keep pace with his rising blood sugar levels. And with every increase, he gained more and more weight. When I first saw this man, he was taking 100 units of insulin daily and had put on 100 pounds!

Bill was in bad shape. But it was not his diabetes but his iatrogenic obesity—which was clearly caused by insulin therapy—that triggered most of his health problems. My treatment plan was simple. I stopped his insulin completely and started him on a proper diet, exercise program, and targeted nutritional supplements. It took several years, but he ultimately lost the extra weight and his blood sugars normalized.

In addition to insulin, which is taken by one in four people with type 2 diabetes, two classes of oral diabetes medications (sulfonylureas and thiazolidinediones) cause weight gain. Other problematic drugs include antihistamines, alpha and beta blockers (used primarily to lower blood pressure), and steroid hormones (corticosteroids), as well as some oral contraceptives and drugs to treat gastroesophageal reflux disease (GERD). Psychotropic drugs are particularly risky. Anticonvulsants are associated with increased weight, as are all classes of antidepressants, including the popular selective serotonin reuptake inhibitors (SSRIs, which include Paxil, Prozac, Zoloft, and Lexapro). Prescribed to 1 in 10 Americans, antidepressants cause a gain of 10 pounds or more in a quarter of those who take them.

Even more worrisome are antipsychotic medications. In a study of children and adolescents on a variety of these drugs, the average weight gain was 1 pound to 1½ pounds per week.[18] Other studies have noted even more dramatic gains in adults—in some cases, more than 100 pounds! These medications also elevate blood lipids, blood pressure, waist circumference, and other markers of metabolic syndrome and increase the risk of diabetes. Furthermore, although they were originally used to treat bipolar disorder and schizophrenia, antipsychotic drugs are increasingly prescribed to children and adults with eating disorders, obsessive-compulsive disorder, tics, aggressive behavior, and severe anxiety.

I also want to mention that gynecomastia (enlarged breasts in men) may be caused by a number of prescription drugs, including antiandrogens used to treat prostate cancer, some HIV medications, Proscar, spironolactone, Valium, tricyclic antidepressants, digoxin, calcium channel blockers, and some ulcer medicines and antibiotics.

Not all medications in all these therapeutic groups are linked to weight gain, but you do need to make sure that the drugs you're taking are not among them. Rest assured that for most of these "fattening" meds, there are safe, natural alternatives.

IS POOR SLEEP MAKING YOU FAT?

Let's add one final and very important item to the list of underlying issues that may be hindering your weight loss efforts: inadequate sleep. As Americans' waistlines have steadily expanded over the past few decades, the duration of our nightly sleep has shrunk. Fifty years ago, we averaged 8½ hours of sleep per night. Today, we get fewer than 7 hours—and an impressive amount of scientific research suggests that this is a pivotal factor in our epidemic of obesity.

Researchers from the United Kingdom performed a meta-analysis of the international literature on sleep duration and weight. Data on more than 634,000 people from around the world, ranging in age from 2 to 102, showed clear and consistent links between duration of sleep and obesity in children and adults.[19] And the impact is significant. According to a study published in *Pediatrics,* kids between the ages of 4 and 10 who get the least amount of sleep are four times more likely to be obese than their peers who get proper rest.[20]

Sleep is a time of recovery and restoration, memory processing and energy consolidation, rest and rejuvenation. It is an important part of our circadian rhythms, the 24-hour cycles of physical, behavioral, and biochemical changes common to virtually all living species. Endocrine activity also follows the circadian clock, so it's not surprising that interrupted sleep affects key hormones. The trouble actually starts even before we go to bed. When the sun sets and darkness falls, the pineal gland in the brain secretes melatonin, the hormone that regulates circadian rhythms and tells your body that it's time to slow down and get ready for sleep. Yet electric lights have blurred the boundary between day and night, with dramatic effects on melatonin release. Many experts believe that melatonin suppression contributes not only to our collective insomnia but also to our increasing problems with obesity and metabolic syndrome.[21]

Short sleep duration and frequent nighttime awakenings disturb other hormones as well. Levels of ghrelin, a hormone that signals hunger, increase while leptin, which tells the brain when we've eaten enough, decreases. So in addition to causing daytime fatigue and low energy, poor sleep messes with the hormonal cues of appetite and satiety, making us more likely to overeat and store fat. Cortisol, another hormone associated with weight gain, also rises with the stress of sleep deprivation.

I understand that these days there's a lot to lose sleep over. People are working longer hours than ever to make ends meet, and there is no shortage of issues to lie awake and worry about. But we also allow sleep thieves such as television, smartphones, and laptop computers into our bedrooms. A 2011 survey conducted by the National Sleep Foundation found that 72 percent of teenagers and 67 percent of 19- to 29-year-olds sleep with their cell phones![22] If they receive texts and calls at the rate my kids do, no wonder they're not getting enough sleep.

You cannot control all of these variables, but do what you can to ensure that you and your family get enough rest. Turn off those devices that keep you connected 24/7. Make your bedroom a sanctuary for sleep. Dim the lights in your home in the evening. Avoid caffeine later in the day, and refrain from stimulating activities in the hour or so before bedtime. If you need extra help, don't turn to sleeping pills, which are addictive and, particularly in older people, linked with falls and cognitive impairment.[23] Instead, try some of the safe, natural over-the-counter sleep aids we use at the clinic. (See "Supplements to Help You Sleep.")

Finally, if you're having a hard time losing weight, talk to your physician about getting tested for sleep apnea. Sleep apnea is the periodic cessation of breathing during sleep caused by relaxation of the soft tissues in the throat, which then block the airway. It's a very common condition that goes undiagnosed in the majority of affected individuals. After all, who's going to run to the doctor because they snore? But sleep apnea is a very serious problem that upsets circadian rhythms, prevents the deeper stages of sleep, and dramatically increases the risk of metabolic syndrome, diabetes,

SUPPLEMENTS TO HELP YOU SLEEP

✔ Supplemental melatonin, taken at bedtime, re-creates the natural nighttime rise in this "sleep hormone." It helps you fall asleep and stay asleep throughout the night. Melatonin is also useful for jet lag, and it's a potent antioxidant that protects against disease.[24]

✔ Valerian *(Valeriana officinalis)* is a popular sleep aid in Europe. This herb has a mild sedative effect, plus it increases levels of gamma-aminobutyric acid (GABA), a neurotransmitter that calms the brain and helps relieve anxiety. Valerian has been shown in clinical trials to be as effective as sleeping pills but without the drugs' adverse side effects.[25]

✔ L-theanine is derived from green tea, which is renowned for its soothing effects. It boosts alpha wave activity in the brain, which results in a sense of relaxation, and works on GABA pathways to tone down anxiety.[26]

✔ Suggested doses of these natural sleep aids are 1 to 3 milligrams of melatonin, 250 to 500 milligrams of valerian, and 200 milligrams of L-theanine. They may be taken individually or in combination formulas 30 to 60 minutes before bedtime.

heart disease, and other serious conditions. Sleep apnea is more an effect of obesity than a cause, as discussed in Chapter 2. However, because it upsets nighttime hormonal cycles, it can also make losing weight an almost insurmountable struggle. Treatment will not solve obesity overnight, but it will give you a fighting chance of regaining control of your weight and other important aspects of your health.

IT'S MORE THAN WHAT YOU EAT

As you can see, weight gain and obesity aren't just about overeating and underexercising. They are complex, multifaceted conditions, and you may need to investigate a number of potential triggers and contributors. I again urge you to rule out these hidden problems that may be holding you back. Once they're corrected and you're working with a clean slate, you'll find the mini-fast with exercise to be the easiest, most rewarding weight loss program you've ever attempted.

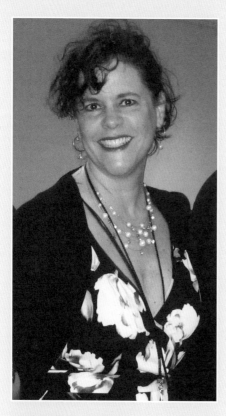

After: After dropping 2 dress sizes, Galen's confident and in control.

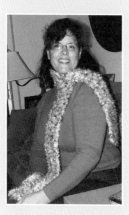

Before: For years, Galen answered "the siren call of sweets" and rode the weight-gain roller coaster.

Galen Clayton: "For the First Time, I'm in Control of My Weight"

Galen Clayton has struggled with her weight for as long as she can remember. By the time she was 9 years old, she weighed more than 100 pounds. Throughout high school, Galen managed to maintain a more or less normal weight. Pretty and outgoing, she had lots of friends and was voted homecoming princess her senior year. Yet she had what she calls "an abnormal relationship with food." She was always on one diet or another, and her favorite was simply not eating. Furthermore, there was the siren call of sweets, especially York Peppermint Patties, which Galen kept in the freezer and snacked on whenever she let her defenses down.

The next 20 years were a roller coaster of gaining and losing, gaining and losing, with weight swings ranging from 15 to 50 pounds. Then 2009 arrived, and for Galen it was a pivotal year. In the course of 3 months, her mother had a severe stroke and her daughter lost her job and moved back home. Then both of Galen's parents and her aunt died—and she got the "good news" that her divorce was final. Once she got through all this and was still standing, she knew that it was time to take control of her life, and that included her weight.

Galen made dramatic changes to her diet. She began a self-imposed sugar detox by eliminating all sweets and foods with more than 4 grams of sugar per serving. It was a 3-month process that was so hard that Galen said she would "rather have gone through a divorce again!" Once that was over, she began cutting out fried foods, bread, and pasta and continued without her nemesis, sugar. In their place, she ate more lean protein and vegetables. She also started working out twice a week with a trainer who specialized in a "super-slow" weight-lifting technique.

Then she heard about the mini-fast with exercise study we were conducting at the Whitaker Wellness Institute, and she jumped at the chance to participate. Because she was already exercising and paying attention to her diet—and, as she says, she "takes orders well"—Galen was a perfect study subject. She cut out breakfast, met with her trainer on Mondays and Fridays, worked out with a Pilates DVD on Wednesdays, and walked a couple of times a week. She also took the supplements we recommended to facilitate fat burning and curb her appetite. After 12 weeks, Galen had lost 10 pounds, which may not sound all that impressive until you realize that it was 10 pounds of fat! She also lost nearly 4 inches around her waist and dropped two dress sizes.

Today, Galen is a walking advertisement for this program, and she never hesitates to share her experiences with anyone who comments on how great she looks and the confidence she displays. "Now that I've won the sugar/carb war, I am free," she says. "For the first time since I was 9 years old, I'm in control of my weight and my life."

CHAPTER 9

YOU'VE LOST WEIGHT. NOW WHAT?

It is not the mountain we conquer but ourselves.

—SIR EDMUND HILLARY

Y ou've lost weight. You feel great, you look fabulous, and your health has improved in myriad ways, some of them obvious and others that will pay dividends in years to come. So what do you do now? By all means, celebrate. This is a significant milestone, and you've earned all the kudos you can get. Go out and treat yourself. Sleep in. Take a couple of days off.

But be careful. Anytime we achieve a personal goal, there is a temptation to sit back and rest on our laurels. The last thing you want to do now is regain the weight you've lost, but that's exactly what happens to far too many folks. Their well-deserved break in their routines stretches out to 2 weeks, a month, and more. They tire of waking up early and start to slack on their exercise. They decide that "just a little breakfast" is okay and become less vigilant about their diets in general.

If you have never lost weight, only to regain it, you may have a hard time understanding how anyone could work so hard for something, then let it slip away. It's really no mystery. To return to my original premise of why so many of us are overweight or obese, it's simply human nature. We are naturally attracted to calorie-dense foods and genetically driven to eat up when such foods are available. We are also hardwired to conserve energy, which is why it's so easy to get out of the exercise routine.

This is the reason the majority of successful losers revert to their old habits and end up where they started—overweight and unhappy about it. Therefore, now more than ever you need to stay focused. Losing weight is just the beginning. Keeping it off is the name of the game.

A JOURNEY, NOT A DESTINATION

The path that brought you here cannot be forgotten once you've arrived. You must stay on it and make it part of your life. You may be able to take slight detours or slow your pace, but you need to keep on going. The mini-fast with exercise is something you *do*, rather than a regimen that you *did* for a period of time. Weight maintenance has to become part of your daily routine. It shouldn't be an obsession, but you cannot allow it to become an unimportant triviality you dabble in whenever you feel like it. You need to make the healthy, positive habits you've developed permanent lifestyle changes.

The requirement to stay the course isn't unique to the Mini-Fast Diet. In Chapter 1, I told you about the National Weight Control Registry (NWCR), a project spearheaded by researchers from the University of Colorado and Brown Medical School. Since 1994, the NWCR has gathered information on more than 5,000 men and women who have lost weight and kept it off. The average loss was 66 pounds, and the mean duration of weight maintenance was 5½ years.

To accomplish their weight loss goals, virtually all of these people changed their diets and increased their activity. And in order to stay slim, they have continued to keep their fat and calorie intakes down and their exercise up. Nine out of 10 walk or otherwise exercise for an hour a day on average. Three-quarters weigh themselves at least once a week. Nearly two-thirds limit their weekly TV time to fewer than 10 hours. (In the interest of full disclosure, I have to tell you that 78 percent also eat breakfast.[1] To revisit my thoughts on that, see Chapter 4.) In other words, once they hit their target weights, they did not go back to their old behaviors but kept up the positive habits that allowed them to lose weight in the first place.

MINI-FAST MODIFICATIONS

What is the next stage in the mini-fast with exercise program? The same as the last one. Just as there was no "induction" phase, there are no "pre-maintenance" and "maintenance" phases. You just keep on doing what you've been doing: fasting in the morning, doing aerobic exercise during the fasting period, and eating sensibly the rest of the day. However, that doesn't mean you can't experiment with modifications to the regimen, if desired.

Mark McCarty, the researcher who originally came up with the mini-fast with exercise program, had, as I told you in Chapter 3, a "eureka moment" while traveling in Japan some 20 years ago when he realized that, during his entire visit, he had seen only one fat person, and that was a man at the airport who may well have been

CONNIE LIVES THE LIFESTYLE

I want to tell you about someone very close to me who is a perfect example of what I'm talking about—my wife, Connie. Connie grew up on a farm near a small town in Nebraska. Her family raised corn and wheat and had a huge produce garden, and they had more than 1,000 head of livestock. One of the reasons she has such a great work ethic and is so down-to-earth is because from a very young age, she and her eight brothers and sisters (you read that right—nine kids!) had to help out with the chores required to keep the place running. Connie is the only one of her siblings who left Nebraska. She is also—and I don't say this to be unkind because they are great people—the only one who doesn't have a weight problem.

I mention this only to make it clear that Connie is not endowed with skinny genes. Like everyone else in her family, she has a tendency to put on weight. In high school she weighed 20 pounds more than she does now, and she's since given birth to five children. (When she went to her 20th high school reunion some time back, no one recognized her.) But she made a decision years ago that she would never be heavy again, and she's stuck with it.

Ever since I've known her, Connie, who is now in her mid-fifties, has looked great. Yes, I'm prejudiced, but I'm not the only one who thinks so. Part of her attractiveness is her personality. She's very high energy; she's never met a stranger; and she's one of the kindest and most generous people I've ever known. But she's also cute as can be and has a great figure—which she earns the hard way.

As I've mentioned, Connie is an exercise enthusiast. In addition to walking and jogging with me, she works out with a personal trainer twice a week and spends time on a stairstepper at the house on the days that she doesn't train. She weighs herself daily, and if she gains more than a pound or two, she modifies her diet. Like most everyone else, Connie loves to eat, but she watches her portions and is able to say no when she needs to. And since we started the mini-fast with exercise—which she absolutely loves—she feels she has more leeway in what she eats the rest of the day.

Again, I'm telling you about my wife only to illustrate that anyone can keep a handle on their weight. All it requires is focus, determination, and a willingness to do what it takes.

arriving from elsewhere. He figured out that it was the Japanese's low-fat diet—not intense exercise or carbohydrate restriction—that was responsible for their nearly uniform leanness.

How does this apply to you? Once you get down to your ideal weight, of course you should continue to mini-fast, exercise, and refrain from overeating. However, if you keep your overall caloric and fat intake at a moderate level, you won't be replacing your fat stores, and you'll be less likely to regain weight, regardless of whatever else you do. In other words, you may be able to liberalize your diet to some degree, but bear in mind the caveats about dietary fat as well as total caloric intake.

Other tweaks to the program you could consider, once you reach your ideal weight, include exercising for shorter or less frequent sessions, say three times a week for 40 minutes versus four times for an hour, or swapping one day of aerobics with a strength-training, muscle-building program. Nevertheless, 3 days of aerobic exercise per week should be your absolute minimum. You can also try exercising outside your mini-fasting period once or twice a week.

Note that I said "experiment with modifications." This means try them and see if they work for you—and the only way you'll know is to monitor yourself with the scale, tape measure, mirror, and other suggestions from Chapter 7. If you are able to maintain your optimal weight while easing up a little on your diet or exercise, good for you. If not, get back on the original program immediately.

BE HONEST WITH YOURSELF

The advantage you have now, compared with when you started the mini-fast with exercise, is that you know you can do it. You have firsthand experience skipping breakfast and exercising regularly, and you understand that, although it takes some discipline, it eventually becomes routine. You realize that you really haven't missed those second helpings and unhealthy foods you've been turning down.

Always be mindful of the most gaping pitfall for anyone who has lost weight: putting it back on. Stay focused by stepping on the scale or otherwise tracking your weight regularly, and if you start to regain, nip it in the bud. Above all, be honest with yourself. Are you really keeping your energy intake and expenditure in balance? Whatever you do, do not get lackadaisical and squander everything you've worked for, because if you do, you'll be back on that thorny old path you left behind, and you certainly don't want to go there again.

"FEELING THE WAY I DO IS ALL THE MOTIVATION I NEED"

Bob Ewing came to see us at Whitaker Wellness with a primary complaint of atrial fibrillation, but like many of our patients, he also needed to lose some weight. So he started on the mini-fast with exercise. He began exercising 7 days a week, walking, cycling, and lifting weights. He also cleaned up his diet and switched to mostly protein, vegetables, and fruit. He does admit to missing breakfast sometimes, but he figures it's a small price to pay.

That's because a year after starting on this program, Bob had lost 30 pounds. His energy level is up; he feels better than he has in some time; and his friends and family notice the difference as well. As for motivation, he says: "Feeling the way I do is all the motivation I need to stay on the Mini-Fast Diet. It's now part of my daily routine, and I'm in for the long haul."

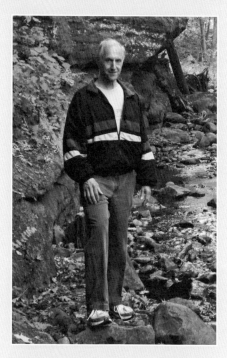

Bill Barbic, a lifelong natural "mini-faster"

Bill Barbic: A Natural Mini-Faster

In addition to my print newsletter, I write a weekly e-newsletter. In response to an article I sent out about the mini-fast with exercise, I received an e-mail from Bill Barbic. My inclusion of Bill's story may seem a little unusual because he didn't lose weight on the mini-fast. Nevertheless, although he'd never even heard of this program, he's essentially been on it for years. I've had feedback from a number of people with similar experiences who are longtime adherents to the particulars of the program, and they all have one thing in common: They are slim, fit, and have never had a weight problem. These natural, lifelong mini-fasters are a testament to the long-term efficacy, safety, and tremendous benefits of the Mini-Fast Diet. Here are Bill's comments.

"I believe in, and practice, a holistic, integrative approach to health that uses the best of the allopathic and naturopathic approaches. The former seems superior in diagnosing and treating trauma; the latter in treating chronic conditions and prevention. I also believe in the power of the mind-body-emotion connection. Although I seek information from a wide variety of sources, I place a great deal of faith in the principle of individuality and ultimately listen to my body and go with my logic plus instincts.

"After reading Dr. Whitaker's e-mail on the mini-fast with exercise, I was struck by how similar it was to a routine I have been on more or less my entire adult life. Since I am usually not hungry when I get up in the morning, I just have black coffee. I start by doing a little review of the prior day, and plan the new day and beyond. I also read something educational and/or inspirational.

"Midmorning every day, I do a combination of exercises that include flex, strength, and some aerobic for 40 to 45 minutes while I channel-surf the news. I do not have my first meal until mid- to late morning or near lunch, again depending on what my body tells me. I usually eat lean protein and low-glycemic carbs (as recommended by the mini-fast plan) for my meals. After lunch I study, write, and do office work. Sometime in the afternoon, I jog about 20 minutes 5 days a week, always before supper. Supper varies with my schedule and social situation, but I try to keep it healthy. I do not smoke or drink alcohol, but I do like desserts and indulge to a point.

"This has worked for me for many years. I am 68 years old and in good health, with a BMI consistently around 23 to 24."

PART III

Exercise and Diet Strategies

Exercising in the mornings works great for me. If I wait, I always manage to come up with some excuse for not doing it. And because I have had good results on the mini-fast, I am more motivated than ever to work out regularly.

—B.B.

My favorite part of this program is that I don't have to make major compromises when it comes to what I'm eating. This is important to me because . . . I knew I wouldn't be able to stick with a diet that didn't allow hamburgers, steak, and the like, and I attribute my success to the fact that I don't feel restricted in my food choices.

—MICHAEL CARNEY

CHAPTER 10

EXERCISE FOR MAXIMUM FAT BURNING

People say that losing weight is no walk in the park. When I hear that, I think, "Yeah, that's the problem."

—CHRIS ADAMS

Exercise is a pivotal part of the Mini-Fast Diet. But I want to say up front that it's also one of the biggest stumbling blocks of this program. It's not that the exercise required is particularly hard or time-consuming. I mean, who can't walk or spare 40 minutes a few times a week? But most people just don't do it.

The 2010 edition of *Health, United States*, the Centers for Disease Control and Prevention annual report released in 2011, revealed some dismaying statistics. Fewer than 20 percent of

Americans get the recommended amount of weekly exercise, and more than a quarter don't exercise at all! It's even worse in the Southern and Appalachian states, where nearly 30 percent do nothing even remotely physically active during their leisure time.[1] (Not coincidentally, these regions have the highest rates of obesity and diabetes.) Our kids, especially teenagers, aren't stepping up either. Just 1 in 10 high school students gets adequate exercise[2]— but a quarter of teens have at least one soda or other sugary drink every day.[3]

We need a wake-up call. Everyone, including the nearly 100 million Americans who don't exercise, knows the benefits of physical activity. But knowledge obviously isn't enough to motivate most people to lace up their running shoes. So let's look at the flip side of the coin: the dangers of *inactivity*.

THE DANGERS OF INACTIVITY

Inactivity doesn't mean sitting on the couch staring into space, napping, and whatnot. The sedentary "activity" that ties up most of our leisure hours is "screen time." And although Americans watch an average of 3 to 4 hours of TV per day, it's not just television. Screen time also includes video games, Internet surfing, texting, and spending time on social media sites—sedentary diversions that, unbelievable as it may seem to younger people, didn't even exist not so long ago.

I understand their allure. Heck, I too get sucked in by TV to a degree I never did in the past. When I was a kid, we had the three network channels, and we watched them on a fuzzy little screen. To see a movie, we had to go to a theater and buy a ticket, and the closest thing we had to video games was "20 Questions," which was inspired by an old TV show. Today, no matter what your interests—sports, history, fashion, cooking, nature, music, film, games, other people's lives—there are compelling programs you can watch and interact with 24 hours a day.

But our infatuation with these sedentary pastimes is taking a toll on our health. In a 2011 study, researchers in Scotland evaluated the impact of screen-time entertainment on the cardiovascular health of 4,500 men and women. They found that the people who spent at least 2 hours of their daily leisure time parked in front of a TV or a computer were more than twice as likely to have a heart attack or other cardiac event. Those who spent 4 or more hours were 50 percent more likely to die![4]

Excessive screen time also contributes to weight gain. Obviously, if you're lounging around, you're burning fewer calories. Furthermore, research demonstrates that we tend to eat more when we're sitting in front of a screen. In the Scottish study, the "recreational sitters," as the researchers called them, had higher BMIs, cholesterol, C-reactive protein (a marker of inflammation), and other metabolic risk factors. In children, excess TV and computer time is linked not only with obesity but also with high blood pressure, poor sleep, inattention, and, in infants and toddlers, delayed language development. Inactivity also increases the risk of diabetes, stroke, osteoporosis, Alzheimer's disease, dementia, erectile dysfunction, cancer, and premature aging.[5] You can't control every risk factor for obesity and these other health challenges, but you *can* be more physically active.

WHY TIMING MATTERS

Any activity you can fit into your day is a boon to your health, and I strongly encourage it. For the mini-fast with exercise, however, timing matters. As I mentioned in Chapter 1, the scientific literature on exercise and weight control suggests that, although physical activity is essential for weight maintenance and prevention of further gain, exercise alone is an ineffective therapy for people who are trying to lose weight. This is largely due to the fact that exercisers tend to eat more.[6] That was certainly the case with me, before I learned about the mini-fast with exercise. I used to eat like a horse after working out. I'd just burned a lot of calories, so I liked to think it didn't matter. Anyway, didn't I deserve a "reward" for my efforts?

This program is different. It doesn't spare you the "work" of working out, but because it's done at a time when you are primed for fat burning, you will lose weight—which makes all the time and effort that exercise entails worthwhile. To reiterate the point that I've been making throughout this book, eating before exercise and/or drinking carbohydrate-rich sports drinks during your workout gives your body a lot of glucose to burn for energy. That's great if you're an endurance runner—you need all the carbs you can get. But your goal in weight loss is to burn stored fat, and that will never happen in the presence of glucose. In short, carbohydrates trigger a release of insulin, which shuts off fat burning and promotes fat storage.

In order to selectively burn fat, you need to exercise when you're fasting and you have no fresh carbohydrates in your system. The first thing in the morning is ideal because you've been fasting all night and your glycogen (carbohydrate) stores are running low.[7] Exercising at this time exhausts your remaining glycogen, so your body turns to burning fat for energy. And you will continue to burn fat until you eat again. If you are unable to exercise in the morning, you can still mini-fast and exercise. Just avoid eating—especially carbohydrates—for as long as possible (at least 2 hours) prior to exercise and continue fasting for several hours afterward.[8] (See Chapter 5 for details on various mini-fast schedules.)

MODERATE AEROBIC EXERCISE FOR OPTIMAL FAT BURNING

Now let's talk about the most effective types of exercise. Fat burning is at its most efficient when you're doing moderately paced aerobic activities. Aerobic exercise works your legs and other large muscle groups, boosts your heart rate and gets blood pumping through your vascular system, increases your oxygen consumption (aerobic means "with oxygen"), and heats up your body temperature and causes you to work up a sweat. This requires energy, which is extracted from biochemical reactions involving oxygen, carbohydrates, and fats in the mitochondria of the cells. When it's done in the fasting state, prolonged aerobic exercise tamps down insulin production, mobilizes fat, and turns on fat burning, which persists for as long as you continue to fast.

Intensity. Studies suggest that exercising in the 60 to 80 percent of maximum heart rate range is optimal. (See "Your Optimal Fat-Burning Exercise Intensity.") This is somewhat counterintuitive. You'd think that more intense exercise would really turn up the furnace, but very high-intensity activity actually has the opposite effect and appears to reduce the absolute amount of fat burned.[9, 10] To burn more stored fat, increase your duration rather than your intensity.

Duration. I recommend that you exercise for at least 40 minutes per session. If you're pressed for time, working out for 20 to 30 minutes is better than nothing. Of course, when you're getting started, you should begin at a lower intensity and a shorter duration and build up gradually as your endurance and strength increase.

Frequency. As for the number of sessions per week, the more often you exercise and activate your fat-burning mechanisms, the faster you'll see results. Four days a week is great, 5 is even better, and 3 is the absolute minimum. After you hit your target weight, you can decrease your exercise frequency, if desired. However, in order to maintain all that you've worked so hard to achieve, you must keep it up. Everyone should be physically active a minimum

YOUR OPTIMAL FAT-BURNING EXERCISE INTENSITY

Fat burning is at its most efficient when you're doing moderately paced aerobic exercise. You should be able to feel like you're getting a workout—heart pumping, lungs taking in more air, muscles working, body sweating—but you should also be able to carry on a conversation. If you find yourself gasping for breath or you feel beat to a pulp, ease up a bit.

A more scientific means of monitoring your intensity level is to figure out your target heart rate, check your pulse periodically while exercising, and pick up or slow down your pace to stay in the optimal fat-burning range. To determine your target training heart rate, first calculate your maximum heart rate in beats per minute. To do this, subtract your age from 220. If you are 25 years old, your max is 195; if you're 45, it's 175. The optimal heart rate for fat burning is 60 to 80 percent of maximum. To compute your personal training range, multiply your maximum heart rate by 0.6 and 0.8. This will give you the number of heartbeats per minute for the most advantageous exercise intensity. Here are some examples:

35 years old: Maximum heart rate: (220 − 35) = 185; 60 to 80 percent (185 × 0.6 and 0.8) = 111 to 148 beats per minute

40 years old: Maximum heart rate: (220 − 40) = 180; 60 to 80 percent (180 × 0.6 and 0.8) = 108 to 144 beats per minute

The easiest place to take your pulse is the carotid arteries, on either side of your neck between the jaw and the collarbone. Stop exercising, and, using your index finger or first two fingers and a watch with a second hand or a digital readout, count the number of beats in 6 seconds (one-tenth of an hour) and add a zero. Say you count 13 beats. Your heart rate for a full minute (13 × 10) is 130, well within the desired range. If you're out of shape, aim for the lower end, and as you become more fit, bump it up to the higher end of your target range.

of 3 days per week. I also suggest that, if at all possible, you skip no more than 2 days between sessions. There will be weeks when life gets in the way and fitting in your scheduled exercise just isn't feasible. Don't worry—just do better next week.

IN PRAISE OF WALKING

Walking is the most popular form of aerobic exercise, and for good reason. It's convenient, it requires no training or special equipment, and it can be modified to suit the needs of everyone from beginners who are completely out of shape to seasoned exercisers. Race walking—which humorist Dave Barry once described as "walking like a dork"—is even an Olympic sport.

Do not underestimate the value of this most basic type of exercise. It's unfortunate that we've lost touch with our "inner walker." If we spent more time walking throughout the day, rather than jumping in our cars to run the shortest of errands, we probably wouldn't be in the shape we are today. America's suburbs and strip malls, along with lengthy commutes, have made walking as a mode of transportation almost obsolete, but it has also lost its allure as a pleasurable activity. Even in this book we're treating it as if it's a chore that you have to make yourself do and "squeeze into" your day.

But walking has benefits beyond the physical. As the Danish philosopher Soren Kierkegaard said: "Above all, do not lose your desire to walk. Every day I walk myself into a state of well-being and walk away from every illness. I have walked myself into my best thoughts, and I know of no thought so burdensome that one cannot walk away from it." Many of my patients can attest to this. Carla calls her morning walks her "time to talk to God." Bob finds that they "clear his head." Jean, a writer, uses the time to organize her day and often comes up with solutions to passages she was struggling with. Harold, who is blessed to have great trails nearby, gets his requisite daily dose of nature. Others use their walks to listen to music, inspirational or educational programs, or audiobooks on an iPod or MP3 player.

Walks can also be social. "The true charm of pedestrianism," according to Mark Twain, "does not lie in the walking, or in the scenery, but in the talking. The walking is good to time the movement of the tongue by, and to keep the blood and the brain stirred up and active; . . . the supreme pleasure comes from the talk." Connie and I often start off our day with a walk. Not everyone is lucky enough to have a spouse they can exercise with—or enjoy talking to—but this is one of our most pleasurable hours of the day. We talk about the kids and the office, the day's schedule, and the usual gossip everyone engages in. We bounce ideas off each other, and when I have an upcoming speech, she lets me use her as a sounding board. The more we talk, the faster we walk, and the quicker the time goes by.

Finally, walking can be an enjoyable pastime. Whenever I travel, I get to know new places by exploring on foot. A few years ago, Connie and I took a "working" European cruise (it wasn't much work—I gave a few talks on various health topics to fellow cruisers). In every port, we got up first thing in the morning, disembarked with a vague itinerary, and started walking. Honfleur, Gibraltar, Lisbon, Barcelona, Cannes, Monte Carlo—we must have logged 5 miles in each of these places. We'd stop for coffee, lunch, or a glass of beer or wine and occasionally pop into museums, shops, and whatever else interested us, but mostly we walked. As a result, we have a sense of familiarity with these cities that we wouldn't have had otherwise.

Recreational walking doesn't have to be so exotic. You can explore unfamiliar areas or revisit favorite parts of your own community. Nature trails make for wonderful walks, even if you have to drive to get to them. You can also build your walk around a destination. A couple of my wife's friends meet every morning at a Starbucks about midway between their houses. They have coffee, catch up on things, and then walk back to their respective homes.

WALKING AS A MEDICAL THERAPY

At the Whitaker Wellness Institute, we encourage our patients, especially those with diabetes, to take a 10-minute walk after meals to help clear glucose out of the bloodstream. We also give a pedometer to everyone who participates in our Back to Health Program. During these 1- to 3-week programs—which consist of physician evaluation, testing, education, and treatment—patients stay at a nearby hotel, but their therapies and appointments are at the clinic 0.8 mile away. Although we have a shuttle service that runs between the hotel and clinic every half hour, we encourage patients to walk.

To promote this activity, we use the most powerful of motivators: competition. Every week we give out prizes to the people who clock the most miles on their pedometers. The awards are nothing special—just books and vitamins. The real prize, of course, is the realization of how easy it is to maintain a walking program and the recognition of its tremendous health benefits. But you'd be surprised at how competitive people get when we turn walking into a "race." These folks really get into it!

Here's just one example. When Ed Schneider of Grafton, Ohio, arrived at the clinic, he was so weak and tired that winning a walking contest was out of the question. Nevertheless, he put on his pedometer every morning and gave it a shot. The first day he totaled just 1,213 steps. But as he underwent various therapies at the clinic and regained his strength and energy, he increased his pace. At the end of his 2-week stay, Ed's record high was 14,160 steps in a single day, and his total was an impressive 104,328 steps—more than 81,000 of them in the second week alone. The average person covers 1 mile in 2,000 steps, so Ed walked a little more than 40 miles that second week, or nearly 6 miles a day. If he kept it up, he could log more than 2,000 miles in a year!

I wrote about the contest in my newsletter and challenged readers to track their steps for 3 weeks. Again, all I had to do was say the words *contest* and *prizes,* and the entries poured in. One subscriber, Beverly Meyers, is director of Sizzling Seniors, a program she started in Saratoga, California, in 1989 to help people stay active through fun, aerobic dance routines. Beverly suggested that her classes participate in this challenge, and we had more than 20 entries from this group alone. The overall winner was John Hansen of Canby, Oregon, who took 424,782 steps in 3 weeks. Actually, this is par for the course for John. A regular walker for years, he averages an incredible 8.7 miles a day, 5 days a week—and it pays off. He has no significant health problems and takes no prescription drugs, which is extremely rare for a man in his seventies.

This contest provided great feedback on the benefits of walking. Aaron Neureuther of Houlton, Maine, reported how walking had a major impact on his health following a six-vessel heart bypass surgery. He averaged 3 to 6 miles per walk and felt better and stronger every day. Richard Lynch of Des Moines, Iowa, said that walking helped keep his blood sugar under control. Gary Baxter of Melbourne, Florida, credited walking with lowering his blood pressure, and Donald Harrison of Buffalo, New York, related how a regular walking program plus diet modifications resulted in a weight loss of 80 pounds!

We also received excellent suggestions on how to fit in, and stick with, exercise. Richard walked the three blocks from his

PACE YOURSELF WITH A PEDOMETER

Pedometers are both a reality check as to how much (or how little) movement you actually get in a day and motivation to become more active. First, the reality check. A 2010 study compared pedometer readings of Americans with those of residents of several other countries and found that, when it comes to walking, we're really lagging. Americans averaged a little more than 5,100 steps a day—fewer than 5,000 steps is considered sedentary—versus more than 9,600 for Australians and Swiss. And we wonder why their obesity rates are 16 and 8 percent, respectively, while ours is 34 percent.[11]

Now for the good news: Pedometers really do increase activity. Researchers at Stanford University and the University of Minnesota, Minneapolis, reviewed data from 26 clinical trials that evaluated the benefits of pedometers. They monitored activity levels in more than 2,700 overweight, sedentary individuals, some of whom used pedometers, while others served as controls. The researchers found that, compared with those in the control groups, study participants who used pedometers increased their daily walking distance by about 27 percent, or an extra 2,100 to 2,500 steps. In other words, they walked an extra mile-plus a day! Over the 18 weeks of the average study, pedometer users also had improvements in blood pressure and weight.[12]

Most people walk 1,000 to 3,000 steps during the course of their daily activities, going to and from their cars, walking around the house, etc. If you get that many steps just hanging out, imagine how many you could chalk up by taking the stairs, parking in the far reaches of the parking lot—and walking for 40 minutes as part of the mini-fast with

home to his workplace and took his dogs for lunchtime strolls. (Dogs are a terrific incentive to exercise.) Gary recruited a neighbor to join him for 45-minute walks 5 days a week. Anna walked for half an hour on her lunch break, and Amelia jogged around the park after dropping her daughter off at preschool. The point I'm trying to make is that, whether you're mini-fasting or not, we all need to seize every possible opportunity to incorporate more activity into our lives.

exercise program! At a moderately brisk pace, the average person can walk at least 3 miles, or 6,000 steps, in an hour.

A reasonable pedometer goal is 10,000 steps per day. If that sounds intimidating, it's easier than you may think. Elizabeth, a patient of mine who wore a pedometer for several weeks, reported that when her job required intense computer work and she didn't have time to do much else, she averaged around 3,500 steps. But on the days she spent outside with her kids, shopping, and running errands, she racked up 10,000 to 13,000 steps. And a busy day full of housework and chores plus a fast-paced walking session resulted in more than 15,000 steps.

You can also use a pedometer to help you gauge your exercise intensity. Researchers at San Diego State University used pedometers to monitor the oxygen uptake and heart rates of study participants as they walked on a treadmill at various speeds. To reach the intensity for optimal health benefits—the target heart rate we talked about earlier in this chapter—the men needed to take an average of 92 to 102 steps per minute and the women, 91 to 115. The researchers concluded: "To meet current guidelines, individuals are encouraged to walk a minimum of 3,000 steps in 30 minutes on 5 days each week. Three bouts of 1,000 steps in 10 minutes each day can also be used to meet the recommended goal."[13]

Pedometers are inexpensive and easy to use, and they're widely available in sporting goods stores, drugstores, and online.

BEYOND WALKING

Walking isn't for everyone. Jogging and cycling are also perennial favorites, as are elliptical gliding, stationary biking, stairstepping, aerobics classes, rowing, and swimming for people who go to a gym or have exercise equipment at home. (Recent research suggests that cycling burns less fat per hour than exercises that require you to support your weight, such as walking, jogging, etc.[14]

CAFFEINE AND SUPPLEMENTS BOOST EXERCISE ENDURANCE

Before heading out the door to exercise, I always drink a cup or two of coffee and take Ketosis Essentials, one of the optional nutritional supplements in the mini-fast with exercise program.

Caffeine decreases reliance on glycogen, mobilizes fatty acids, and stimulates fat burning. According to the 2010 position statement of the International Society of Sports Nutrition (ISSN), "Caffeine is effective for enhancing sport performance . . . when consumed in low-to-moderate doses." In addition to increasing endurance, caffeine improves insulin sensitivity. Insulin resistance is at the heart of metabolic syndrome, the cluster of conditions that include abdominal obesity, hypertension, and lipid and blood sugar problems. Coffee also dramatically reduces the risk of type 2 diabetes.

As for the popular notion that caffeine is a diuretic that causes dehydration, the ISSN further states, "The scientific literature does not support caffeine-induced diuresis [excessive urination] during exercise, or any harmful change in fluid balance. . . ."[15] In summary, pre-exercise caffeine is a three-way winner: It wakes you up and may thus improve motivation; increases endurance; and provides much needed hydration during exercise.

Ketosis Essentials is a combination of hydroxycitric acid (HCA), a botanical extract from *Garcinia cambogia;* two amino acids, carnitine and glycine; and chromium, a trace mineral. Carnitine is required for the transport of fatty acids into the mitochondria, the power plants of the cells where energy is produced. HCA boosts fat burning and curbs appetite, which improves endurance and makes mini-fasting easier to handle. Glycine serves as a precursor to compounds necessary for energy production. And chromium improves insulin sensitivity. The ingredients in Ketosis Essentials have a synergism that facilitates the burning of stored fat and increases exercise endurance, plus it reduces appetite and makes the fasting period more tolerable. To use, mix one scoop in water and drink prior to exercising. You may take another dose a few hours later if you're having difficulty fasting.[16] (To read more about this supplement, see Chapter 5.)

However, cycling is easier on the knees and hips and is a reasonable option if you're dealing with joint pain or injury.) Other home-based aerobic activities include mini-trampolines and a wide range of exercise DVDs—*P90X* is one that will kick your you-know-what—and video games such as Wii Fit.

I understand that doing the same thing day in and day out, especially when you're flying solo, can get a little boring. Fortunately, many recreational and group activities are aerobic in nature. Hiking, skating, martial arts, power yoga, and singles tennis, racquetball, and other racquet sports are all aerobic activities, as are basketball, soccer, and other team sports that don't involve a lot of standing around. In fact, most any activity will suffice, provided that it requires you to use the large muscles of your legs and arms and increase your cardiovascular workload—and that you do it for long enough and at a sufficient intensity. You can turn an hour in the park with your kids or grandkids into an aerobic workout by playing tag, tossing or kicking a ball around, and playing games that involve brisk walking, running, and jumping. The goal is to make it fun so you'll actually *want* to exercise.

WALKING + JOGGING = WOGGING

When I first got back into exercise after an embarrassingly lengthy break, I walked. After a few months, I began interspersing it with jogging. I didn't really plan to add in running—it just happened rather spontaneously as my endurance improved. I'd slog up a hill, for example, then slowly jog down. On flat stretches I'd pick a landmark 100 to 200 feet out, jog that distance, and resume walking. There was nothing scientific about it. I called it "wogging" (walking plus jogging) and thought I'd coined a clever word until I realized that someone had beat me to it.

Although wogging is higher impact than walking, it's an activity that most people can do, especially as their conditioning improves with regular walking. If you're like me, you may already do it without putting much thought into it. And if you're young and in pretty good cardiovascular shape, you may need to add some jogging to step up your intensity in order to maintain your target heart rate.

Wogging requires no special equipment, other than a pair of running shoes. But because jogging involves more impact than walking, it's worth investing in decent shoes. You may be able to walk in Keds, but you need more cushioning and stability when you jog to absorb the shock of pounding the pavement and take the stress off your joints.

As with walking, wogging can be done anywhere—indoors on a treadmill or on a track at the gym in inclement weather. However, if possible, I suggest that you seek out grass, dirt roads, jogging trails, school running tracks, and even blacktop roads. These surfaces have more "give" than concrete sidewalks and thus absorb shock and reduce stress. When you wog, you're going to cover more ground than you do when you're just walking, so plan your routes accordingly. There's nothing wrong with wogging around the block multiple times, but it can get boring. Mixing it up helps reduce the monotony factor that contributes to slacking off.

12-Week Wogging Program

Wogging isn't rocket science, but for those of you who like a little structure, here is a 12-week progressive wogging program designed by Rodale senior director of fitness and health and marathon champion Budd Coates. This program is actually designed to get you in shape to run a 5-kilometer race (3.1 miles). Although that's not exactly the purpose here, signing up for a 5-K is a great idea because it motivates you to exercise regularly in preparation for the big day.

If you're able to walk comfortably at a relatively brisk pace for 30 minutes, you should be able to undertake a progressive wogging program. However, if you have any medical issues or if you're over age 50 and haven't been exercising at all, I suggest that you get clearance from your doctor before beginning. The only equipment you'll need, in addition to reasonably good shoes, is a watch with a second hand or a digital readout.

Start each session with a 5-minute walk to warm up your muscles and end each session with another 5 minutes of walking to cool down. A little gentle stretching—with an emphasis on gentle—of your leg muscles is also recommended. When first starting out, try to give yourself a rest day between workouts while your body adjusts to the higher intensity. On your off days, simply walk or do interval training that involves some strengthening exercises.

Also, if you feel you're not ready to move to the next level, don't. Repeat a week, or alter it to where you feel comfortable. There's no rush to get to 30 minutes of running—and if you never get there but still alternate between running and walking, that's fine, too. Remember, this is just a guide.

WEEK	JOG: WALK (MINUTES)	REPS	TIMES PER WEEK
1	2:4	5	4
2	3:3	5	4
3	5:2.5	4	4
4	7:3	3	4
5	8:2	3	4
6	9:2	2 (then jog for 8 more minutes)	4
7	9:1	3	4
8	13:2	2	4
9	14:1	2	4
10	14:1	2	4
11	30: no walk	1	4
12	30: no walk	1	4

STRENGTH TRAINING IS ALSO IMPORTANT

All this emphasis on aerobic exercise in no way diminishes the importance of resistance, or strength, training. If you're a woman, your primary goal with this kind of exercise, which is specifically aimed at strengthening and building up the muscles, may be shapely arms, a flat belly, and a firm butt. Men, you may be after a six-pack and bulging biceps. These are laudable objectives, but resistance exercise also provides a number of perks. In addition to augmenting aerobic exercise's positive effects on insulin sensitivity and bone density, strength training enhances weight control.[17, 18]

Your basal metabolic rate (BMR), which, as we discussed in Chapter 4, is the number of calories you burn at rest to fuel respiration, heartbeat, blood circulation, body temperature maintenance, and other vital activities, depends on several factors, and one of them is your muscle mass. The more lean muscle you have, the higher your BMR and the more calories you burn, even when you're sleeping. The reason men and younger people have higher BMRs than women and older people is because, on average, they have more muscle. This segues into another, very important benefit of resistance training. As we get older, we tend to lose muscle. This phenomenon, known as sarcopenia (which means "vanishing flesh"), is a significant contributor to the frailty, limited mobility, and increased risk of falls in elderly people. The only way to stave off and reverse age-related muscle atrophy is to build muscle through resistance exercise.

All of the activities we've discussed so far will increase the muscle mass in your legs, but the upper body is often neglected in people who concentrate solely on aerobic exercise. And while strength training isn't required as part of the mini-fast with exercise program, I strongly suggest that you work in a couple of

MORNING WALKS A BOOSTER SHOT— AND A FAMILY AFFAIR

Sarah Dela Cruz is another top-notch employee at the Whitaker Wellness Institute who participated in our mini-fast with exercise study. Here's what she had to say:

"I cannot say I've really 'struggled' with my weight because I never really worried too much about it. I have Crohn's disease and had a bad flare-up in 2008, during which I lost more than 10 pounds and was pretty sick. But I gained it back and wanted to lose 15 to 20 pounds, so I decided to try the mini-fast with exercise.

"I exercise almost every day with 30 minutes of brisk walking. Because of my Crohn's, my diet is pretty good—I eat mostly fish, veggies, walnuts, and dried fruit. I do get hungry in the mornings occasionally, and sometimes I go ahead and eat.

"I've only lost about 5½ pounds, but my waist has shrunk considerably, and I've gone down one clothing size, which goes to show you that weight isn't everything. I plan to stay on the mini-fast with exercise. I like taking brisk walks early in the morning. It feels like you're getting a booster shot early on to get you going for the rest of the day, and it makes me feel more energetic and alive. Another plus is that it has become a family affair. My husband and daughter walk with me!"

sessions per week. You can do this on your own with pushups, pullups, situps, hand weights, barbells, or your own body weight. (See the home-based program beginning on page 210.) If you are inexperienced but serious about weight training, I suggest you join a gym and/or sign up for a handful of sessions with a personal trainer who will help you learn the proper techniques.

15-MINUTE HOME STRENGTHENING EXERCISE PROGRAM

There's no place like a gym or a health club with its variety of weights and exercise machines for strength training. However, memberships cost money, and getting there and back takes time. I've had enough requests over the years for a quick, at-home, no-equipment-required program that I've come up with a simple but effective set of strengthening exercises. To avoid injury, start slowly and build up gradually, and make sure that you warm up with 5 minutes of walking or gentle stretching—or do this routine after your mini-fast exercise. For most of these exercises I've recommended that you do two sets. However, if you're in a hurry, do just one set, or concentrate on your upper body one day and your lower body or core the next.

Exercises to Build Up Your Core

Not so long ago, most of us didn't even know we had a "core." Today, with all the Pilates and yoga studios, not to mention the emphasis on toned abs, exercises abound to strengthen the 29 muscles in the trunk and pelvic area that make up your core. In addition to defining your abdominal muscles, core exercises strengthen the back, improve posture, and reduce the risk of back pain and injury. A strong core also creates stability in your center of gravity, which is indispensable for improving athletic performance and, for older people, maintaining optimal function and independence. Here are some core exercises to do at home.

TWISTING CRUNCHES

Lie on your back with your legs up, knees bent, and lower legs parallel to the floor. Clasp your hands behind your neck with your elbows out to the sides. Tightening your abdominal muscles and pressing your lower back to the floor, raise your shoulder blades off the floor as you twist your right elbow toward your left knee. Return to the center, shoulder blades still raised, and twist to the other side. Do 15 repetitions, alternating sides. Lower your head and upper back down to the floor. Rest and repeat.

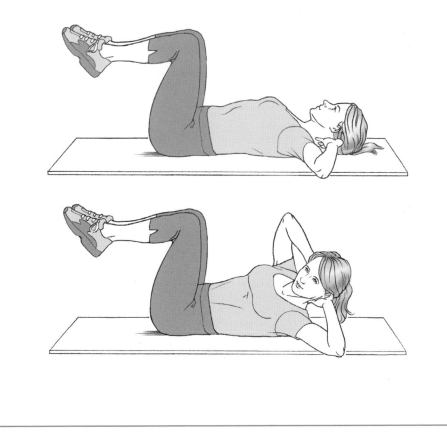

BRIDGES

Lie on your back with your knees bent, feet flat on the floor about hip-width apart and close to your buttocks. Keep your arms straight at your sides with your palms facing down. Slowly lift your pelvis so that your hips and lower back are off the floor while your upper back and shoulders remain in place. (You'll be using your back muscles.) Hold for 5 to 10 seconds, then slowly lower your hips back down to the floor. Relax and repeat 10 times. Rest and do another set of 10.

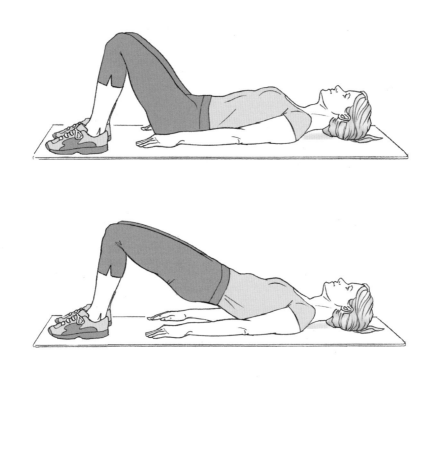

SUPERMAN

Lie on your stomach with your chin or either cheek against the floor. Stretch your arms out in front of you and, tightening the muscles in your buttocks and lower back, raise your outstretched arms, chest, and legs off the floor. Hold for 10 to 15 seconds, then relax. Repeat for a total of three sets.

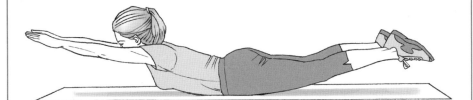

Toning and Strengthening Your Arms and Shoulders

While you technically can "buy" a great chest, stomach, and derriere with implants and liposuction, you have to earn toned arms and shoulders the old-fashioned way, with exercises such as the following:

PUSHUPS

Lie on the floor facedown, toes tucked under, with your hands about level with your shoulders. Keeping your stomach muscles tight and your body in a straight line, slowly straighten your arms and raise yourself off the floor, then lower yourself back down so you're hovering inches above the floor. (Modified pushups, with your knees on the floor and your body straight, are perfectly acceptable.) Do as many pushups as you can in 1 minute, rest, and repeat.

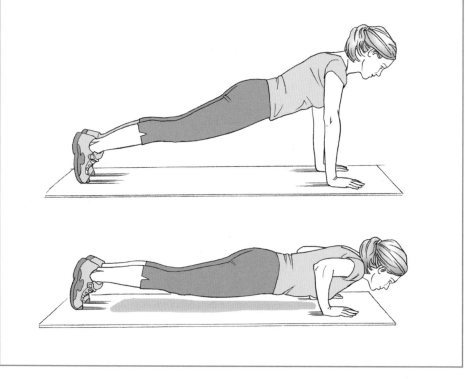

ARM CIRCLES

Stand with your feet hip-width apart and raise your arms out to your sides, parallel to the floor. Keeping your elbows and wrists straight, posture erect, and shoulders back, make small clockwise circles with your hands, about a foot in diameter, for 30 seconds. (Increase to 60 seconds in each direction as you get stronger.) Reverse direction, and make counterclockwise circles for another 30 seconds. Relax and repeat.

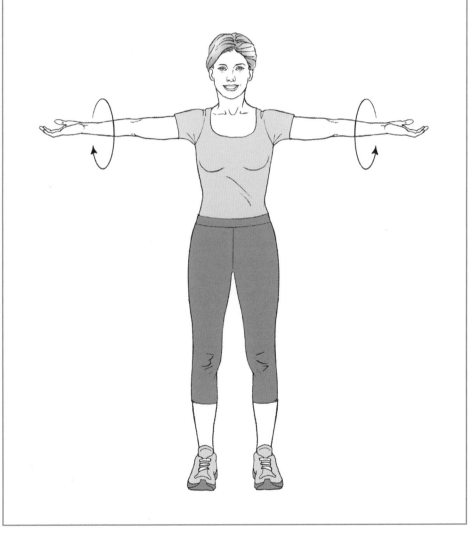

WALL PUSHUPS

Stand facing a wall, about 6 inches more than arms' length away. Extend your arms straight toward the wall at shoulder level and parallel to the floor. Leaning forward, rest your palms against the wall, adjusting your hands a little, if necessary, to whatever feels comfortable. (You'll be supporting your weight as you lean forward.) Now slowly bend your elbows and move your chest toward the wall, keeping your body straight and taking care not to bend at the waist. Slowly push back to the original position. Do a total of 15 repetitions. Rest and repeat.

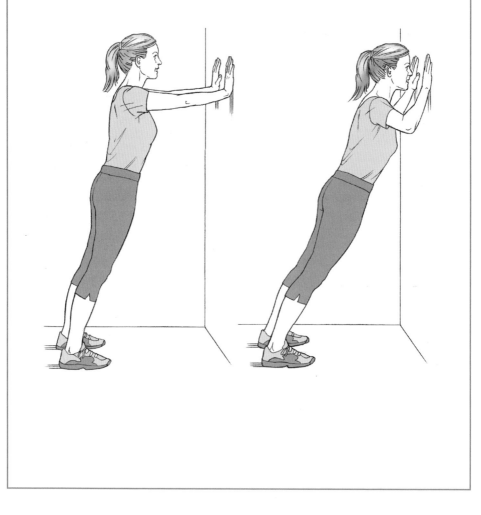

BICEPS CURLS

Stand with your feet hip-width apart and your arms at your sides. Bend your right arm at the elbow until your forearm is parallel to the floor, palm facing up. Place your left hand on top of your right wrist or open palm. With your elbow tucked into the side of your waist, move your right forearm up so that your hand is near your right shoulder, then move it straight down toward your right thigh. At the same time press with your left hand to create as much resistance as you can handle. Do 15 repetitions, then switch sides. Rest and repeat.

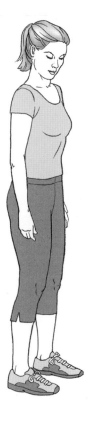
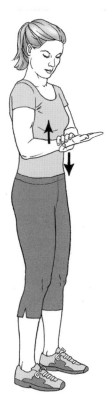

Keep Your Lower Body Strong and Fit

With all the aerobic activities you're doing on the mini-fast with exercise program, your lower body muscles are getting a pretty good workout. Here are some additional exercises that target the glutes, hamstrings, quadriceps, and calf muscles.

SQUATS

Stand in front of a chair or near a wall with your feet hip-width apart and your toes pointing out slightly. Holding on to the chair or wall, if needed for balance, slowly bend your knees, leaning your upper body forward a bit, until your thighs are almost parallel to the floor. (You'll be in a near seated position.) Pause, then slowly return to a standing position. Repeat 10 times. Rest, then do another set of 10.

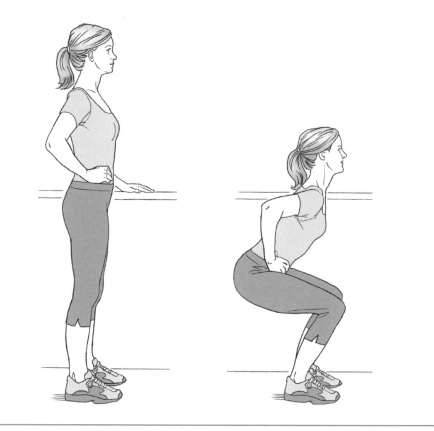

LUNGES

Stand with your feet hip-width apart, hands on your hips or holding on to a wall or chair, if needed for balance. Step forward with your right foot, and position yourself so that your right knee is bent at a 90-degree angle directly over the ankle and your thigh is parallel to the floor. (Your left leg may be slightly flexed for balance.) Hold for a few seconds, then bring your left leg up to meet the right. Repeat on the other side, stepping out with your left leg. Repeat 10 times on each leg, alternating sides. Rest and perform another set of 10.

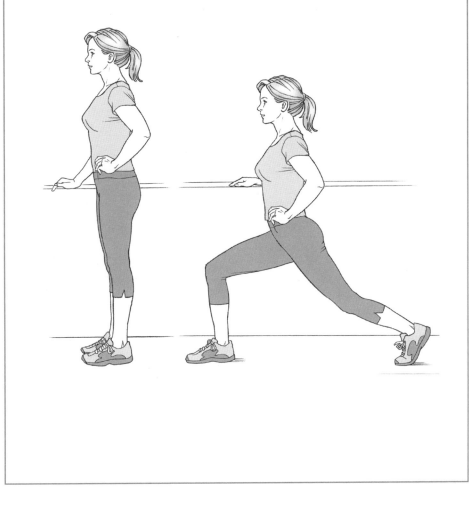

QUAD STRENGTHENERS

Sit in a chair with your back straight. (Place a rolled-up towel under your knees for support, if desired.) Engaging your back and abdominal muscles, slowly lift your feet until your legs are straight in front of you and parallel to the floor. Hold for 10 seconds, then slowly lower your feet to the floor. (If it's more comfortable, you may alternate legs.) Do 10 repetitions. Relax and repeat.

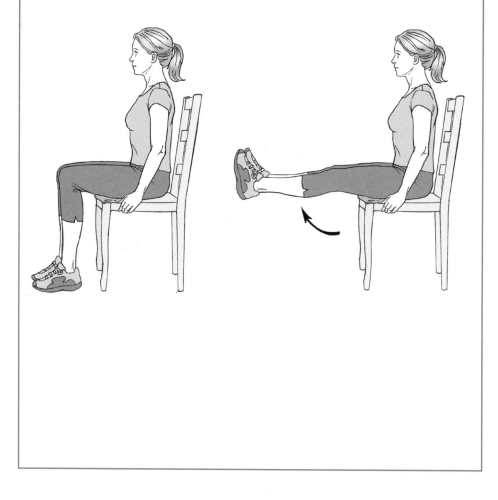

STEP-UPS

Stand at the bottom of a step or stairs. With your toes facing forward, place your left foot on the first step. (If you want a greater challenge, place your foot on the second step.) Holding on to the handrail and keeping your posture erect, straighten your left leg and bring your right foot up to the step. (More experienced exercisers: With a straight knee, lift your right leg as far behind you as you can before putting it on the step.) Lower your right foot back to the floor, followed by your left leg. Do the same thing on the other side, leading with your right foot. Repeat 10 times on each side, and alternate leading with either leg. Rest and complete a second set of 10 repetitions with each leg.

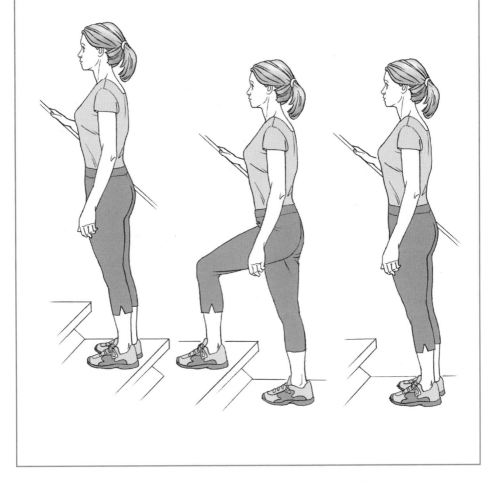

CALF RAISES

Stand up straight near a wall or chair. Slowly raise yourself up on your tiptoes as high as you can, steadying yourself with the wall or chair if needed. (This is also a great balance posture.) Hold for 10 seconds and slowly lower yourself back down. Pause and repeat 10 times. Relax and do another set. (You can make this exercise more difficult by squatting as you remain on your toes.) For variation and to work different areas of the calf muscles, do additional sets with your heels together and toes pointed out, and with your toes pointed inward and your heels out.

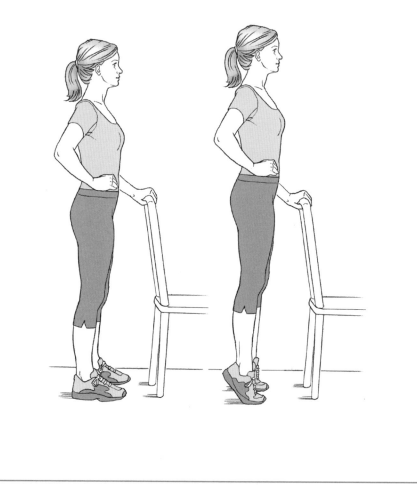

PUT ONE FOOT IN FRONT OF THE OTHER

I wish I could offer an alternative program that didn't involve exercise, but I can't. There are no shortcuts to healthy, sustainable weight loss. Aerobic exercise performed in the fasting state is the single most efficient method of turning on fat burning, kick-starting ketosis, and getting rid of unwanted fat stores. Resistance exercise builds muscle, which tones the body, enhances strength, boosts basal metabolism, and helps keep weight off.

Exercise requires intention and effort, and it's something that you and only you can do. You must make the commitment. You have to muster the motivation to get started. And it's up to you to figure out what it takes for you to stay on track. I understand how easy it is to put exercise on the back burner. I've heard all the excuses (and used many of them myself): "I'm too tired," "I'm too sick," "I'm too out of shape," "It's too boring," and that old standby, "I'm too busy." I've provided a number of strategies and tools to refute these justifications for not exercising. In Chapter 6, "Staying on Track," I've given suggestions for fitting exercise into a busy schedule and hectic mornings, ideas for finding or creating a support group to keep you focused on exercise, and a surefire motivational technique called instant willpower.

There's an old saying that goes, "A journey of a thousand miles begins with a single step." These wise words are a spot-on description of embarking on an exercise program. You've made the decision to lose weight, and you understand what's required. All that's left for you to get started is to put one foot in front of the other. Keep your eye on your goal—a trimmer physique, better health, and more energy and vitality—and get moving!

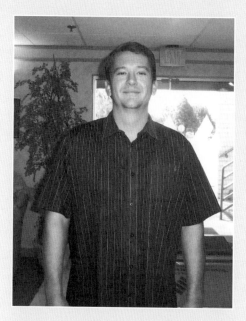

Brian after losing 40 pounds on the mini-fast with exercise

Brian Shook: "I'm at a Weight That I Hadn't Seen in More Than 20 Years"

Brian Shook has been working at Whitaker Wellness on a consultant basis for 8 years. He's our computer guy, and we don't know what we'd do without him. He's a bright, conscientious young man who not only participated in the mini-fast study we conducted at the clinic, but he was our "biggest loser." Here's what Brian had to say about the program.

"Since I was a kid, I've had weight issues. I remember getting a physical to play football when I was 14, and I already weighed 190 pounds. Over the years I've tried a few diets, and I'd lose maybe 10 pounds, but I'd usually gain them back. When I heard about the mini-fast study, I was intrigued because it was so different, and I decided to participate. My goal was to lose 25 pounds.

"I got very serious about exercise and did 45 minutes on an elliptical machine every morning. I can't say it was easy exercising every day, but I loved doing it first thing in the morning because then I didn't have to think about it again. I also found that it really helped with stress during the day. I also give a lot of credit to the supplements, which I took every day. Everyone I talked to who was not having a lot of success with the program was either not taking the supplements or not exercising right when they woke up.

"Skipping breakfast was easy for me because I prefer to just drink coffee in the morning. But I made a serious effort to stay away from sugar. I have a really bad sweet tooth and used to eat a lot of sweets before I went to bed. I also cut back on carbohydrates and ate mostly protein and salads.

"When I started on this program last summer, my goal, as I said, was to lose 25 pounds. Given my history, I figured that was pretty ambitious. But I lost 5 pounds the first week, which made it really easy to stay motivated. Within 4 months I lost 31 pounds, and was down to 174. After a year I lost 40 pounds, and went from a 36- to 38-inch waist to a 32 to 34. I actually felt like I lost too much weight, so I moved to a different exercise program and I'm working on building muscle. Instead of doing all cardio workouts, I alternate between cardio and weights. I've deliberately gained some of it back by putting on muscle.

"For a guy like me who has always been overweight and never been able to get the pounds off, the idea of intentionally gaining weight is kind of funny. But it's proof that this program works. At age 35, I'm at a weight now that I hadn't seen in more than 20 years."

CHAPTER 11

NOT A DIET, JUST SENSIBLE EATING

My doctor told me to stop having intimate dinners for four. Unless there are three other people.

—ORSON WELLES

The beauty of the mini-fast with exercise program is that it isn't a diet per se. Yes, you are skipping a meal every day and, in the process, cutting out considerable calories. But as I've said before, you're not required to count calories, figure out grams and percentages of fat, measure protein portions, or eliminate carbohydrates or any particular foods. Many people get good results without making major modifications in their usual food choices. But good results are virtually a slam dunk if you're sensible about what you eat.

I understand that "sensible" is highly subjective. A serving that one person considers moderate is minuscule to another, and there are people who seem to have convinced themselves that a pizza-and-fast-food diet is acceptable. In an effort to provide some clarity, in this chapter we'll discuss two key components of sensible eating: the quantity and the quality of the foods you choose.

THE AVERAGE AMERICAN DIET

Before we get to our discussion of what you *should* eat, let's look at what Americans actually *are* eating. In 2011, the Consumer Reports National Research Center polled more than 1,200 people nationwide about their diet practices and eating habits. Ninety percent of survey participants defined their diets as "somewhat," "very," or "extremely" healthy. But were they?

They claimed to be making several healthy food choices, with 50 to 60 percent eating whole grains such as brown rice instead of white rice, limiting their intake of sugars and fats, and consuming five or more servings of fruits and/or vegetables per day. (The surveyors didn't exactly question the honesty of respondents but did note that, according to a 2010 Centers for Disease Control and Prevention [CDC] report based on interviews with 421,000 Americans, fewer than a third consumed two daily servings of fruit, including juice, and just a quarter ate three or more servings of vegetables, which they consider the bare minimum.[1])

On the other hand, 43 percent also admitted to having at least one soda or other sweetened drink per day—and that includes a quarter of those trying to lose weight and a third who labeled their diets very or extremely healthy. The most popular vegetables were lettuce and tomatoes, which nearly three-quarters said that they ate at least once a week, followed by carrots, potatoes, broccoli, corn, and peppers, which were eaten weekly by 50 to 60 percent. Kale, Swiss chard, spinach, sweet potatoes, beans and peas, and other nutrient-dense vegetables were way, way down on the list.[2]

Most telling, this group was a pretty typical cross section of the country in terms of weight. Approximately 35 percent were of normal weight, 36 percent were overweight, and 21 percent were obese. (I'm not sure about the other 8 percent; they were unaccounted for.) If these people truly were eating as well as they thought they were, they would have been much closer to their ideal weight. You don't become overweight or obese eating a "somewhat," "very," or "extremely" healthy diet.

This leads us to one of two conclusions: Either these people were fudging a little in their responses or they really don't understand what a healthy diet is. I'm not saying they were dishonest, but as any doctor can tell you, patients tend to gloss over their bad health habits and embellish their good ones, just as they do their compliance with recommended therapies such as diet and exercise. Nevertheless, given all the conflicting advice out there, I'm sure that a fair number of people are uncertain as to what actually constitutes a healthy diet.

You'd think that government guidelines would be a reasonably reliable source of information. Every 5 years, the US Department of Health and Human Services (HHS) and the US Department of Agriculture (USDA) team up to create the "Dietary Guidelines for Americans." Their latest iteration, released in 2011 after years of work and untold millions of taxpayer dollars, is essentially a litany of how poorly we're eating and a rehash of recommendations that, considering our current epidemic of obesity, haven't helped in the least.[3]

In a media blitz that featured First Lady Michelle Obama, these agencies rolled out MyPlate, a jazzy new graphic designed to improve Americans' eating habits.[4] It's certainly an improvement over the tired, confusing food pyramid that had been around for years. But like its predecessor, it displays undue influence of at least one special interest group—dairy has a very prominent position. Furthermore, it's way too vague. That plate, which is separated into four sections (fruits, vegetables, grains, and protein) plus a "side" of dairy, could be filled with a skinless chicken breast, steamed broccoli, organic quinoa, and raspberries—or with Colonel Sanders' Kentucky Fried Chicken, mashed potatoes and gravy, a biscuit, and canned fruit cocktail.

Categorizing foods isn't as simple as dividing a plate into brightly colored quadrants—nor are Americans that simpleminded. In every one of these groups, there are good foods and not-so-good foods: foods that quench your hunger and foods that leave you craving more, foods that are a boon to your health and foods that have no place in a healthy diet.

GET A HANDLE ON OVEREATING

I want to make a few comments about *quantity* before we move on to the quality of specific foods. Many of us just eat too much. If you're one of them and you really do want to permanently win the battle of the bulge, you need to come to terms with this once and for all. Gluttony is a harsh term, but it truly does describe how some people eat—and it's a fairly easy habit to acquire.

As discussed in the opening chapter, we have a natural tendency to overeat in order to sock away calories for times when food is scarce, even if those times never come. Furthermore, like other things required for survival of the species, eating is highly pleasurable. Have you ever pushed away from the table, adequately and perhaps even uncomfortably full, and then dessert comes along and you manage to devour an entire serving? Most of us have. The pleasure centers in our brains are overriding our satiety signals. (Note how this phenomenon occurs only with foods rich in fat, sugar, and calories. You've probably never eaten Brussels sprouts or oatmeal to the verge of bursting.)

The point I want to make is that overeating becomes a habit—and habits can be broken, once you put your mind to it. Lewis of

Newport Beach, California, who has lost 16 pounds on the mini-fast with exercise, says: "I've always had a hearty appetite. My wife is a great cook, and I love to eat. I am not much of a snacker, but mealtime is something else. Not only would I eat everything on my plate, but I'd also mop up what she and the kids left on theirs. They used to call me the human garbage disposal. For most of my life, it didn't matter, so I always figured I was one of those lucky guys who wouldn't gain weight. But as I got older, the pounds crept on. I didn't like it, but I didn't change my eating habits either.

"When I decided to do this program, I not only stepped up my exercise and skipped breakfast, but I also decided to try to eat less. When my wife asked me if I wanted seconds, much to her surprise I said no. When we went out to a restaurant, rather than eating all of my dinner plus the half of hers she didn't finish, which I used to routinely do, I tried to stop at half or three-quarters and take the rest home. I wasn't always successful, but some restaurants serve such huge portions that our leftovers are usually enough for at least another full meal. This took some effort at first because I could easily have eaten more. What I discovered was, I wasn't having seconds and sometimes thirds because I was hungry. It was just the habit, expectation, and enjoyment of food. I could still eat the same foods and enjoy them without stuffing myself."

It's time to buckle down and get a handle on the amount of food you consume. I don't care how well you eat or if you exercise 45 minutes every day, weight loss won't happen if you're eating 4,000 calories a day. Training yourself to eat less is really just a question of becoming more conscious of what and when you eat and making a decision like Lewis did to do something about it. Because the mini-fast with exercise requires making changes in your exercise and eating habits, why not go full-bore and work on portion control as well? Here are some suggestions that might help.

PORTION DISTORTION

Our concept of what constitutes normal servings has expanded over the years. Walk into most restaurants and you'll see plates overflowing with enough food to feed two, three, even four people. Take a look at how portion sizes have increased over the past 20 years.[5]

	20 YEARS AGO		TODAY	
	Portion	Calories	Portion	Calories
Bagel	3" diameter	140	6" diameter	350
Cheeseburger	1	333	1	590
Spaghetti with meatballs	1 cup sauce 3 small meatballs	500	2 cups sauce 3 large meatballs	1,020
Soda	6.5 ounces	82	20 ounces	250
Blueberry muffin	1.5 ounces	210	5 ounces	500

Source: Modified from "Portion distortion and serving size," National Heart, Lung, and Blood Institute. www.nhlbi.nih.gov/health/public/heart/obesity/wecan/eat-right/distortion.htm.

At Home

◆ **Enlist your family's help.** If you are fortunate to have someone preparing your meals, ask that person to help you out by serving smaller portions and not offering seconds. Or if you're the chief cook, do everyone a favor and make the transition to more reasonable serving sizes. Lewis's story about cleaning up not only his plate but also those of his family will likely hit home with many parents, so get the kids involved as well.

◆ **Fill half of your plate (or more) with vegetables or salad.** Leafy greens and fresh veggies are great sources of low-calorie, nutrient-dense carbohydrates, so stack your plate high with them. Try to steer clear of croutons, fatty dressings, and cheesy sauces, which add unnecessary calories, and sauté, grill, or roast your vegetables with a little extra-virgin olive oil to keep them on the healthy side.

• **Avoid serving meals "family style."** One surefire way to eat too much is to shovel heaps of food onto your plate from large serving bowls. Dish out single servings and store the leftovers in single-serving portions.

• **Use smaller plates.** Sensible portions can look a little meager on a giant plate. Using smaller plates will ensure you don't feel "cheated" by seeing all that empty space. Studies show that this simple trick really does work.

• **Don't eat in front of the TV or computer.** Being distracted while you chow down makes overeating way too easy. Concentrating on and enjoying your food—not to mention the company of those you're dining with—will make you less likely to overindulge.

• **Eat an apple before lunch and dinner.** If you have a hard time not overdoing it at mealtime, try eating a small or medium-size apple about 30 minutes before lunch and dinner. Apples are a wonderful source of satiating fiber, which not only helps fill you up but also keeps your digestive tract running smoothly. (If you have diabetes, be sure to monitor your blood sugar, as fruit may drive it up.)

• **Eat slowly.** It takes 15 to 20 minutes for satiety signals—the feeling of fullness—to reach your brain. If you eat too quickly, you'll clean your plate and go for seconds before you even realize you're full. Chew food thoroughly, put your fork down between bites, and engage in conversation with others in an effort to make mealtime a little less frenzied.

PORTION GUIDE

To make it easier to visualize what moderate serving sizes look like, here's an easy reference to help you gauge appropriate portions.

4 ounces of chicken or meat = a deck of playing cards or a little more

4 ounces of fish = a checkbook or a little larger

2 tablespoons of peanut butter or cream cheese = a golf ball

1 ounce of cheese = a pair of dice

1 ounce of sliced cheese or deli meat = a DVD

½ cup of cooked rice = a cupcake wrapper

½ cup of cooked pasta = a cupped palm

1 small potato or sweet potato = a computer mouse

½ cup of fruit or vegetables = fingers and knuckles of a small fist

¼ cup of nuts = an adult-size handful

1 cup of chopped vegetables or fruit = a baseball

1 medium-size piece of fruit = a tennis ball

Dining Out

◆ **Skip the bread and chips.** Unless you have exceptional restraint, inform the server that you'll pass on the basket of bread or chips that many restaurants provide. Don't kid yourself. Once that warm, fragrant bread or those tortilla chips and salsa make it to the table, they're history.

◆ **Request substitutions and modifications.** Have all sauces and salad dressing served on the side. Instead of a loaded baked potato, french fries, or a giant scoop of white rice as a side dish, ask for steamed or grilled vegetables, cottage cheese, a side salad, or fruit. Don't be shy about requesting things that aren't on the menu. One of my favorite "off menu" items is a salmon fillet or chicken breast served on a big salad.

- **Share or split orders.** Share an entrée with a friend, or ask your server to split your meal before bringing it to the table. Have half served in the restaurant and the other half wrapped to go. Other tips include making an appetizer or two your main dish or ordering a kid's meal. They may frown upon a 40-year-old eating a kiddie meal, so get it to go and eat it at home.

- **Avoid temptation.** If you know that you can't see a pizza without eating five slices, skip it altogether and opt for a different menu item. Better yet, go somewhere that pizza isn't served.

- **Stay away from all-you-can-eat buffets.** Tables piled high with attractive displays of every type of food under the sun are sure to sabotage even the best intentions.

- **Say, "No, thank you."** "Do you want that supersized?" "No, thank you." "Would you like to order an appetizer or side dish?" "No, thank you." "Would you like to see the dessert menu?" "No, thank you."

- **Don't go out to eat when you're starving.** I realize it sounds silly to eat something before going out to eat, but if you arrive at a restaurant famished, chances are you'll have poorer judgment when it comes to ordering than you might otherwise.

WHAT SHOULD YOU EAT?

We've discussed when you should eat: any time but during your fasting/exercising window. We've discussed how much you should eat: Watch portion sizes and don't pig out. Now let's talk about *what* you should eat.

At my clinic, we use food as medicine. Since 1979, the Whitaker Wellness Institute has treated around 50,000 patients, and virtually every one of them has received a prescription for a therapeutic diet (plus a nutritional supplement program). I do not use the word *prescription* lightly. We literally use nutrition and other safe, noninvasive therapies in place of prescription drugs.

Our diet prescriptions are, of course, individually tailored and vary from person to person and condition to condition. But they all stem from a common philosophy, which is that the best foods for optimal health are those that are closest to their natural state. These are the foods that people have had access to throughout most of human history, foods that the body recognizes and is used to digesting and utilizing for energy, repair, and growth. There may be some debate as to exactly what our prehistoric ancestors ate. Were we primarily hunters or gatherers? We may never know, but one thing we know for sure is that they weren't drinking sodas, eating Twinkies, or dining at McDonald's.

The diets we prescribe at Whitaker Wellness contain a wide variety of plant foods, which are naturally low in fat, high in fiber, and rich in phytonutrients. We include moderate amounts of protein from sources such as wild Pacific salmon, lean chicken and beef, eggs, low-fat and fat-free dairy, and beans and legumes. Processed foods may be convenient, but they're stripped of essential nutrients and loaded with fat, sugar, salt, and other additives. Much of what we eat today would be unrecognizable to someone who lived 100 years ago and was magically transported to modern America, let alone our predecessors from the distant past.

Don't get me wrong—I'm all for convenience. In the next chapter, you'll find recipes created by the Rodale Kitchen that include items such as canned tomatoes, frozen chicken breasts, and prewashed spinach. But you won't find recipes that call for white sugar or margarine. I'm not saying you can never eat these items, but they should not be mainstays of your diet.

Some of you reading this book will opt to follow the 2-week menu plan and prepare the recipes in the following chapter. Others will pick and choose, perhaps substituting healthier versions of favorite dishes. Still others will ignore this section entirely and either eat what you've been eating, perhaps more sensibly, or follow another food plan that works for you. All of these approaches are acceptable. My one and only desire is that you achieve your weight loss goals—and I know you'll reach them much more rapidly if you clean up your diet in addition to following the fasting and exercise regimen.

Enjoy Lean Protein

Protein is an essential nutrient for growth and repair, and its constituent amino acids are the building blocks of enzymes, hormones, and other vital substances. From the perspective of weight control, dietary protein has a number of advantages. Of all the macronutrients, it's the most satiating. Because it fills you up and tides you over, a high protein intake is associated with a reduced overall calorie load.[6] Another benefit of protein is that it actually helps burn calories. Digesting food and absorbing and storing nutrients require energy. This process, called diet-induced thermogenesis, uses up about 10 percent of your daily caloric expenditure. Fat metabolism doesn't take much energy because adipose cells absorb fatty acids with relative ease. Carbohydrate digestion is more involved, but protein is the front-runner by far—it burns up 20 to 30 percent of calories ingested, compared with carbohydrates' 5 to 10 percent, and fat's mere 3 percent or less.[7]

Regimens such as the Atkins diet, which emphasizes more protein (and fat) and less carbohydrate, do tend to perform better early on in head-to-head studies when comparing them with other diets. However, few people manage to stick with low-carb diets over the long run.[8] I am by no means recommending that you cut out carbohydrates, but I do suggest that all of your meals contain some protein. A reasonable amount is a 4- to 5-ounce serving (20 to 30 grams of protein), or a little more if you have a big build. Good sources include fish and seafood, skinless poultry, lean meat, eggs and egg whites, nonfat or low-fat cottage cheese and Greek yogurt, reduced-fat cheese, tofu, and soy and whey protein. (For more options and serving sizes, see page 252.)

Be Smart about Fats

We are naturally drawn to fatty foods; they taste good and are satisfying. But excessive dietary fat plays a significant role in our epidemic of obesity. If someone took a syringe, stuck it in the subcutaneous fat in your buttock, thigh, or abdomen, took out a sample, and analyzed its fatty acid composition, it would give a reasonably clear indication of the kinds of fat you've been eating. If your diet contains a lot of monounsaturated fats, they end up in your adipose tissue. Polyunsaturated, saturated, trans fats—if you eat them, they're there in your fat cells.[9]

I'm telling you this not because I think you should have your fat analyzed but to illustrate how easily dietary fat is stored. Think of your fat cells as large-capacity storage units that readily pick up fats (triglycerides) as they float in the bloodstream. As long as you keep filling them at a pace that outstrips fat removal for energy needs, they keep getting larger and larger. This is an extreme oversimplification, but I want you to understand that if you eat a lot of fat, it will inevitably end up in your adipose cells—replacing the fat that you've been burning off on the mini-fast with exercise.

Once you get down to your target weight, you will likely be able to liberalize your fat intake a bit, provided, of course, that you keep up the fasting and exercise.

I am not advocating a very low-fat Pritikin or Ornish diet, although both plans have been embraced by some of our successful mini-fasters. Like extremely low-carbohydrate regimens, these restricted diets are difficult for most people to adhere to.

DOES ORGANIC MATTER?

I'm often asked what I think about organic food and if it's worth the extra price. I do believe that it's superior, both nutritionally and environmentally. The bulk of the produce in our supermarkets is grown in chemically enriched soils and doused with pesticides, but organic fruits and vegetables are becoming more and more widely available. Not only are organic vegetables and fruits cultivated without chemical fertilizers or insecticides and guaranteed not to be genetically modified, but studies suggest that they are more nutritious.

Most livestock are raised in feedlots or other extremely cramped conditions, given antibiotics to prevent disease and growth hormones to put on weight, and fed unnatural diets specifically designed to fatten them up and bring them to market faster. (If we were all forced to observe this process up close, there would be a lot more vegetarians in this country.) By definition, organic animals live in less stressful environments and have access to the outdoors, are fed organic food, and aren't given prophylactic drugs. Some organizations, such as the Organic Consumers Association, maintain that many of the large commercial organic dairies are simply glorified feedlots and that organic eggs often come from hens that never go outdoors.[10] Nevertheless, the USDA's organic certification program is a step in the right direction. From a health perspective, grass-fed beef is leaner and has a better fatty acid profile than its nonorganic counterpart, and, like organic chickens, eggs, and milk, it's blessedly devoid of hormones, antibiotics, and other drugs.

It's true that organic food costs more, so I suggest checking out food co-ops and farmer's markets to find the best deals. As far as fruits and vegetables go, you may also consider "going organic" only when buying produce that's most heavily treated with chemicals, and

Furthermore, some types of fat are essential for optimal health: omega-3 essential fatty acids in salmon, mackerel, and other fatty fish; and omega-6s in nuts, seeds, grains, and vegetables. Mono-unsaturated fats, which are present in olive oil, avocados, almonds, and hazelnuts, are also recommended. As far as cooking oils go, stick with extra-virgin olive oil or, for dishes in which the taste of olive oil is a little overwhelming, canola oil.

organic is your only option at that point. The Environmental Working Group, a nonprofit consumer protection organization, publishes an annual list based on pesticide tests from the USDA and the FDA. Here are the 2018 results. [11]

The Dirty Dozen (buy organic)

Strawberries	Cherries
Spinach	Pears
Nectarines	Tomatoes
Apples	Celery
Grapes	Potatoes
Peaches	Sweet bell peppers

Clean 15 (with the least pesticide)

Avocados	Mangoes
Sweet corn	Eggplants
Pineapples	Honeydews
Cabbages	Kiwis
Onions	Cantaloupes
Frozen sweet peas	Cauliflower
Papayas	Broccoli
Asparagus	

Steer clear of trans fats, found primarily in partially hydrogenated oils in some margarines, baked goods, snack items, and fried foods. These are the most harmful dietary fats and should be strictly avoided. Go easy on saturated fat, particularly in animal products, as it contributes to insulin resistance and thus to weight gain. Vegans and others who eat a low saturated-to-unsaturated fat ratio are usually lean, even if their diets aren't particularly low in total fat. You don't have to be vegan, but everyone should place reasonable limitations on saturated fat intake by staying away from fatty cuts of beef and pork, poultry skin, whole-fat dairy products, and more than one egg yolk per day. (If you want more eggs, switch to egg whites and eat them to your heart's content.) There is a saturated fat that I encourage, and that is coconut oil. Made up mostly of lauric acid, a medium-chain triglyceride that confers several health benefits, coconut oil lends a unique flavor to sautéed foods and is an excellent substitute for butter or margarine in baking.

Be aware that, in addition to the fat in meat and other animal products, Americans get most of their dietary fat from processed and prepared foods: fried items in restaurants, chips and other snack foods, frozen appetizers and dinners, and all manner of desserts. These calorie-rich, nutrient-poor foods are a minefield for anyone serious about losing weight. The fats you consume should be those that are naturally present in whole foods. In other words, feel free to enjoy nuts, olive oil, salmon, skinless chicken, and some eggs. Dove Bars and french fries—not so much.

Eat Plenty of Low-Glycemic Carbohydrates

Carbohydrates, as you'll recall from our discussion in Chapter 3, are the body's primary energy source. But not all dietary carbs are created equal. From a biochemical perspective, they fall into two basic categories: simple and complex. Simple carbohydrates like fructose and sucrose are made up of one or two sugar molecules, while complex carbohydrates, which we typically think of as starches and fiber, are composed of longer chains of sugars. With the exception of fiber, which passes through the body undigested, all carbohydrates are ultimately broken down in the digestive tract into simple, single-molecule sugars, primarily glucose. Once glucose is absorbed into the bloodstream, its presence prompts the pancreas to secrete insulin, which signals the cells to let it and other nutrients into the cells.

The real difference among carbohydrates is not whether they're simple or complex but what happens once they're eaten—and that's where the glycemic index and load come in. The glycemic index takes into account how quickly a carbohydrate is broken down into glucose and enters the bloodstream. For example, starches in white potatoes are clearly complex, yet they are rapidly converted into glucose. Meanwhile, fructose, as simple a sugar as you can get, barely affects blood sugar. But this is only part of the story. Because the glycemic index is determined by measuring the blood sugar response of a set number of grams of carbohydrate, it doesn't take into account the amount of a particular food that is normally eaten. For instance, watermelon has a high glycemic index, but because it's made up mostly of water, each serving contains a relatively small amount of carbohydrate. Therefore, it has a much less significant effect on blood sugar and a lower glycemic load. Spaghetti, on the other hand, is dense and starchy, so a serving contains more carbs and thus has a higher glycemic load. And baked white potatoes have both a high glycemic load and index.

Glycemic index and load are determined by a number of factors, including the type of starch, the degree to which the food has been processed (the more processed, the higher on the glycemic scale), the amount of fat and fiber it contains (both slow the release of sugar), how finely it has been ground (finely ground grains are higher), and the amount of carbohydrate per serving. As you would expect, most natural foods, including beans, legumes, vegetables, and some fruits and whole grains, are low glycemic, while highly processed foods, sugars, flour, refined grains, and fruit juice are high glycemic. There are some outliers, of course, but they are few and far between.

Why does this matter? Because high-glycemic carbs cause a rapid rise in blood sugar and insulin levels. What goes up must come down, so these spikes are followed by falls, which are sometimes so dramatic that you end up with low blood sugar, or reactive hypoglycemia, which makes you tired, hungry, and irritable. In comparison, low-glycemic carbohydrates are broken down more slowly and take longer to be absorbed, resulting in less dramatic fluctuations in blood sugar and insulin. This translates into a steadier supply of energy, more sustained satiety, fewer blood sugar swings that can cause food cravings, and less stress on glucose- and insulin-dependent metabolic processes.

If you are serious about losing weight and keeping it off, low-glycemic, high-fiber carbohydrates should become a mainstay of your diet—and high-glycemic carbs must take a backseat. Rather than memorizing glycemic values, I suggest that you simply eat more natural foods and fewer processed ones. Feel free to load your plate with unlimited amounts of leafy greens and non-starchy vegetables. Eat modest amounts of fruit, two or three servings per day, and go easy on juice. (If you have diabetes, limit your fruit intake even more, as it can really spike blood sugar.) And don't go overboard on grains. Whole grains are okay, but most of the grains that Americans eat are refined, and refined grains are linked with an increased risk of insulin resistance and abdominal obesity.[12] Enjoy a modest serving (half a cup) of brown rice or quinoa or a

FILL UP ON FIBER

Insoluble fiber, found in whole grains and the skins and outer coatings of seeds, fruits, and legumes, promotes regularity and wards off constipation. Soluble fiber, present in fruits, vegetables, seeds, and grains, helps maintain healthy blood sugar and cholesterol levels. Fiber-rich foods are also quite satiating, so you'll feel full longer after eating and be less inclined to overindulge. Although most people are aware of the importance of fiber, the average daily intake is in the range of 15 grams per day; very few get the recommended 25 to 30 grams. If you're having trouble getting this amount from vegetables, fruits, and whole grains alone, add ¼ cup of freshly ground flaxseed or another source of fiber to your daily diet.

Food	Serving Size	Fiber (in Grams)
100% bran cereal	⅓ cup	9.1
Pinto beans (cooked)	½ cup	8
Artichoke hearts (cooked)	½ cup	7.2
Black beans (cooked)	½ cup	7
Lima beans (cooked)	½ cup	7
Garbanzo beans (cooked)	½ cup	6
Pear	1 medium	5.5
Soybeans (cooked)	½ cup	5.2
Quinoa	½ cup	5
Apple	1 medium	4
Mixed vegetables (cooked)	½ cup	4
Raspberries	½ cup	4

slice of sprouted grain bread, but bagels and white rice are best left alone. (To learn more about the glycemic index and load and the values of specific foods, visit the University of Sydney's searchable database at www.glycemicindex.com.[13])

THE LOWDOWN ON SWEETENERS

On average, Americans consume 22.2 teaspoons of sugar per day. That adds up to 355 calories—20 percent more than we were eating 35 years ago—and it's showing up in our expanding hips and waistlines and increasing blood sugar and blood pressure levels. Regardless of whether or not you are trying to lose weight, there's nothing sweet about all those calories.

The only sweeteners I wholeheartedly recommend are stevia and xylitol. Stevia, extracted from *Stevia rebaudiana,* an herb native to South America, is calorie free, has no effect on blood sugar levels, and is completely natural. Just a few drops of a liquid concentrate or a dusting of powdered stevia is all you need to lend sweetness to any dish. It's the sweetener of choice at the Whitaker Wellness Institute, and if you haven't tried it, you should. Some people find that stevia has an unpleasant aftertaste. If you experience this, try another brand with a high percentage of rebaudioside A, the phytonutrient in stevia with the sweetest and least bitter taste.

Xylitol is a sugar alcohol, and although it isn't calorie free, it is metabolized much more slowly than sucrose (white sugar) and has a low glycemic index and load. It looks and tastes a lot like sugar, and is an ideal substitute in baking or anywhere you'd use sucrose. Although xylitol is completely safe, some people are sensitive to all sugar alcohols, which can cause loose stools and gastrointestinal upset, so introduce xylitol to your diet slowly to avoid potential problems.

The Fructose Fiasco

High-fructose corn syrup (HFCS) has received a lot of bad press in recent years. There's even talk of an "anti-obesity" tax on this ubiquitous product, which has overtaken sucrose as the sweetener of choice in drinks and prepared foods. HFCS certainly deserves its bad rap—but so do other sugars. Sucrose is broken down in the body into 50 percent fructose and 50 percent glucose. HFCS, despite its name, is actually a blend of fructose and glucose, in ratios of 55:45 in soft drinks and 42:58 in foods. From a health perspective, HFCS, sucrose, and most other caloric sweeteners are pretty much the same. They all drive up blood sugar and insulin levels, provide insignificant nutritional value other than calories, and deliver a hefty serving of fructose—which creates problems of its own.

There's nothing wrong with a little fructose. After all, it occurs naturally in fruit, packaged with fiber, vitamins, and other nutrients. But we cannot handle the massive amounts of fructose in sodas, fruit drinks, desserts, and countless other products. Fructose is rapidly taken up by the liver, where it is converted into fat. (The conversion of fructose to fat is far more efficient than with other carbohydrates.) Some of this fat is released into the bloodstream, driving up triglycerides, and some is stored in fat cells. Extra calories from any source contribute to weight gain, but fructose has a special talent for packing on pounds in the abdominal area. And this fat distribution, as you know, is linked with metabolic syndrome, diabetes, and cardiovascular disease. Studies also suggest that fructose consumption interferes with satiety-signaling hormones, which may contribute to overeating and greater weight gain.

A high intake of fructose also raises blood levels of uric acid and increases the risk of gout. It is implicated in nonalcoholic fatty liver disease, which is most common in overweight people with metabolic syndrome. In addition, it's 8 to 10 times more reactive than glucose in terms of initiating the chemical reactions that create advanced glycation end products (AGEs), which are an underlying cause of diabetic complications, cataracts, Alzheimer's, and overall aging.

BEWARE OF ARTIFICIAL SWEETENERS

Many dieters are tempted by the promises of calorie-free artificial sweeteners such as aspartame (NutraSweet, Equal), sucralose (Splenda), acesulfame K (Sunett), saccharin (Sweet'N Low), and neotame (similar to aspartame). What could be better than a zero-calorie sweet fix?

Although these chemical sweeteners are found in thousands of consumer products—from obvious junk food items like soft drinks to "healthy" fare such as yogurt and cereal—they bring no nutritional value to the table. Furthermore, they have checkered safety records. In an article published in the *Journal of the American Medical Association,* Harvard professor David S. Ludwig, MD, PhD, says that artificial sweeteners may actually contribute to weight gain. They mess up the body's natural hunger and weight controls, and because they are so intensely sweet, they may make natural, healthy foods less appealing. He cites studies showing links between a high consumption of diet drinks and a twofold increased risk of becoming overweight or obese. He also notes that daily intake is associated with a heightened risk of metabolic syndrome and type 2 diabetes.

I'm not so naive as to think that everyone will swear off their Diet Coke, Pepsi, or whatever, but if you do indulge, I urge you to do so in moderation. Although Dr. Ludwig admits in his article that artificial sweeteners have received a lot of scientific scrutiny, he calls Americans' unprecedented consumption, especially in diet drinks, "a massive, uncontrolled, and inadvertent public health experiment."[14]

Do your best to avoid not only high-fructose corn syrup but also the excess sugars in sodas and processed foods. If you have a hankering for something sweet, reach for stevia or xylitol.

BEVERAGES CAN BLOW—OR BOOST—YOUR WEIGHT LOSS

In the Consumer Reports Survey discussed at the beginning of this chapter, 43 percent of the respondents reported drinking at least one sugary drink daily.[15] Liquid calories make up approximately 20 percent of the average American's daily caloric intake. Just one of these beverages per day adds up to 50,000 calories in a year. To put this in perspective, a pound of body fat is equal to about 3,500 calories. Therefore, that daily sugary beverage could conceivably add about 15 pounds of weight annually! That's a surefire way to blow any diet.

Sodas, it should go without saying, have no place in a sensible diet. But if you simply must have a soda every once in a while, try Zevia. Sweetened with stevia and erythritol (a sugar alcohol) and available in flavors like cola, root beer, and lemon-lime, Zevia is the only soft drink that I'd even consider recommending. Some grocery chains carry Zevia, or it can be purchased in health food stores or online.

Sports/energy drinks aren't much better. Americans spend billions of dollars annually on these specialty drinks, but if you take a close look at their labels, you'll see that most are little more than "sexy" soft drinks, loaded with sugar and calories. For example, Red Bull, the energy drink that "gives you wings," contains 110 calories and 27 grams of sugar per 8-ounce can. Gatorade, perhaps the most popular sports drink, boasts just 50 calories and 14 grams of sugar per 8-ounce serving—but the average bottle contains about 20 ounces. And though VitaminWater certainly sounds more promising, it has a similar calorie and sugar profile. In fact, in 2009 the Coca-Cola Company (VitaminWater's manufacturer) was slapped with a class action lawsuit alleging that marketing the beverage as healthful was deceptive. While some specialty drinks may be truly therapeutic, the purported benefits of most are overblown and unproven. Unless you are exercising vigorously and sweating profusely, stick with water.

Fruit drinks, more often than not, contain more sugar and artificial flavors and colors than they do actual fruit. If you're going to have juice, make sure that it's unsweetened, no-sugar-added,

100 percent juice, and limit your intake to 6 ounces per day to avoid going overboard in the calorie and sugar departments. Individuals who have metabolic syndrome or diabetes or who want to lose weight are better off refraining from fruit juice altogether. One exception is tomato juice. (Tomatoes are billed as vegetables but they're actually fruit.) At the clinic, we serve Low Sodium V8 juice to our patients. Unlike most other juices, it contains very little sugar, making it ideal for people minding their weight or blood sugar levels. It's also a great source of both lycopene, which protects against cardiovascular disease and some types of cancer, and potassium, a mineral that helps keep blood pressure under control. Stick with Low Sodium V8, as regular tomato juice has a lot of salt.

Water should be your beverage of choice—and it may even help you lose weight. Researchers at Virginia Tech recently found that adults on a reduced-calorie diet who drank about two 8-ounce glasses of water before meals lost more weight than those on the same diet who did not drink water before meals. After 12 weeks, the water drinkers lost an average of 15.5 pounds, compared with 11 pounds for those in the control group.[16] If you're "bored" with water, add a twist of lemon, lime, or orange and a little stevia, if desired. Or try sparkling water (club soda, carbonated water, seltzer water, or soda water). And to remind yourself to drink more, keep water bottles in your car, on your desk, by your bed, and next to your favorite chair.

Coffee is another winner. I sometimes get strange looks when people hear that I view coffee as a health food, but it confers a number of undeniable benefits. It protects against Parkinson's and Alzheimer's, promotes alertness, helps control asthma and alleviate headaches and migraines, and improves insulin sensitivity. Coffee also curbs appetite and increases endurance when used before workouts—which is precisely why the mini-fast with exercise protocol encourages a cup or two prior to your morning workout. (I'd like to clear up the ever-present myth that coffee and other caffeinated beverages are dehydrating. An expert panel concluded in 2004 that caffeine-containing drinks not only do not cause dehydration, but they actually help keep you hydrated.) If you don't drink your coffee black, use a little low-calorie creamer and/or sweetener, but stay away from sweetened lattes, mochas, and other high-calorie coffee drinks. And if caffeine makes you jittery or keeps you awake at night, limit your intake to one or two cups early in the day.

Tea—black, white, or green; iced or hot—is another great option for anyone on the Mini-Fast Diet. If you're not a coffee drinker, have a cup or two of tea in the morning before your workout. In addition to caffeine, tea boasts several health-enhancing ingredients. The best studied is epigallocatechin-3-gallate (EGCG), which is particularly abundant in green tea. EGCG is a potent antioxidant that protects against a multitude of health challenges, including heart disease, Parkinson's, cancer—and obesity. (See Chapter 5 for information on how supplemental EGCG promotes fat burning, curbs appetite, and stimulates weight loss.)

Alcohol can have a place in a weight loss regimen, plus it has a number of health benefits. Used in moderation, alcohol reduces the risk of heart attack, improves insulin sensitivity, helps stave off cognitive decline, boosts bone density, and even promotes healthy weight. But more than one or two drinks a day can have disastrous effects. If you consume alcohol, stick to the recommended serving sizes (5 ounces of wine, 12 ounces of beer, and 1 ounce of hard alcohol), and don't add unnecessary calories by stirring in sugary mixers. If you have a problem with alcohol, avoid it altogether. And never drink during your mini-fasting period. Alcohol will shut fat burning off in a flash.

SALT AND OTHER SEASONINGS

Americans currently consume a whopping 3,400 milligrams of sodium every day—which is 1,100 milligrams more than the recommended daily intake for healthy individuals, and almost 2,000 milligrams more than what is suggested for people with high blood pressure, diabetes, or kidney disease. Because we get most of our sodium from processed and prepared foods, the easiest solution is to cut back on restaurant meals and frozen, canned, packaged, and deli fare.

But there's more than meets the eye to the sodium story. In addition to watching your sodium intake, you should eat more potassium. Balancing your potassium-to-sodium intake, in a ratio of 4:1, not only helps regulate blood pressure but also reduces water retention, which contributes to weight gain. According to a 2010 Dutch study published in the *Archives of Internal Medicine,* the effects of eating more potassium are "of similar magnitude to what can be achieved by lowering sodium intake." The researchers suggested that this could be accomplished by having more potassium-rich vegetables and fruits and replacing sodium chloride (regular table salt)—especially in processed foods, our most abundant source of sodium—with potassium salt.[17]

We've been doing that at Whitaker Wellness for years. In place of regular salt, we mix three parts potassium chloride (Nu-Salt or Morton's Salt Substitute) with one part sodium chloride. Potassium chloride by itself can have a metallic taste, but when it's mixed with a little regular salt, few people can tell the difference. To flavor foods at home, try this potassium-salt combo.

Do not forget the abundance of herbs, spices, and other seasonings to jazz up your food. Tasty options include:

Allspice	Chili powder
Anise	Chipotle peppers
Basil	Cilantro

Cinnamon

Cloves

Coriander

Cumin

Curry powder

Dill

Garlic powder

Ginger

Horseradish

Italian seasoning

Ketchup

Marjoram

Mint

Mrs. Dash

Mustard

Nutmeg

Onion powder

Oregano

Paprika

Parmesan cheese

Parsley

Pepper

Red-pepper flakes

Rosemary

Sage

Salsa

Soy sauce (low-
sodium)

Tabasco

Tarragon

Thyme

Vinegar

Worcestershire sauce

SENSIBLE SNACKING

Smart snacking is an important part of any long-term weight management plan. If you ask most people why they don't stick to diets,
they'll tell you it's because they can't handle being hungry all the
time. My answer is, as long as you're outside your mini-fasting
period, have a snack! Snacking not only satisfies your immediate
hunger but, provided that you select healthy snacks, also reduces
your chances of overeating at the next meal. Notice that I said
"smart" snacking, because what you eat between meals can make
or break your diet.

According to data from a survey published in 2011, Americans get, on average, a quarter of their daily calories from
snacks. The most popular items, in descending order, are alcohol;

(continued on page 254)

HEALTHY FOODS AT A GLANCE

Here's an alphabetized list of a number of healthy foods and sensible portion sizes that you should feel free to eat on a regular basis.

Alfalfa/bean sprouts (unlimited)

Almond butter (2 tablespoons)

Almonds (¼ cup)

Apples (1 medium)

Applesauce, unsweetened (⅓ cup)

Apricots (2–3 whole)

Artichoke hearts (¾ cup)

Asparagus (unlimited)

Avocados (½ cup)

Beef, lean (4 ounces)

Bell peppers (unlimited)

Black beans (½ cup)

Blackberries (1 cup)

Blueberries (½ cup)

Boysenberries (1 cup)

Broccoli (unlimited)

Brown rice (½ cup cooked)

Brussels sprouts (1 cup)

Cabbage (unlimited)

Cantaloupe (1 cup)

Carrots (1 cup)

Cashews (¼ cup)

Cauliflower (unlimited)

Celery (unlimited)

Chard (unlimited)

Cheese, reduced-fat preferred (1 ounce)

Cherries (½ cup)

Chicken (4 ounces)

Cod (4 ounces)

Corn (½ cup)

Cottage cheese, low-fat or fat-free (¾ cup)

Crab (4 ounces)

Cucumbers (½ cup)

Deli meats, low-sodium, low-fat (4 ounces)

Eggplant (1 cup)

Eggs (1 whole per day)

Egg whites (unlimited)

Fruit, canned, water-packed (½ cup)

Garbanzo beans (½ cup)

Grapefruit (½)

Grapes (¾ cup)

Green beans (1 cup)

Ground turkey (4 ounces)

Halibut and other whitefish (4 ounces)

Honeydew melon (½ cup)

Kale (unlimited)

Ketchup (2 tablespoons)

Kidney beans (½ cup)

Kiwifruit (1 whole)

Lettuce (unlimited)

Light cream cheese (2 tablespoons)

Lima beans (½ cup)

Mandarin oranges, canned, water-packed (½ cup)

Mayonnaise (2 tablespoons)

Mushrooms (unlimited)

Mustard (2 tablespoons)

Nectarines (1 small)

Nuts (¼ cup)

Oatmeal, steel-cut or slow cooking preferred (½ cup)

Olives (¼ cup)

Onions (unlimited)

Oranges (1 small)

Peaches (1 medium)

Peanut butter (2 tablespoons)

Peanuts (¼ cup)

Pears (1 small)

Pickles (½ cup sliced or 1 small whole)

Pineapple (½ cup)

Pinto beans (½ cup)

Plums (1 medium)

Pork tenderloin (4 ounces)

Quinoa (½ cup cooked)

Raspberries (1 cup)

Salmon (4 ounces)

Salsa (¼ cup)

Scallions (unlimited)

Shrimp (4 ounces)

Snow peas (1 cup)

Soybeans/edamame (1 cup)

Soy protein (20–25 grams)

Soy sauce, less-sodium (1 tablespoon)

Spinach (unlimited)

Sprouted grain bread (1 slice)

Squash, winter and summer (1 cup)

Strawberries (1 cup)

String cheese (1 ounce)

Sunflower seeds (¼ cup)

Sweet potato (1 small)

Tangerines (1 medium)

Tofu (8 ounces)

Tomatoes (unlimited)

Tortilla (1 small corn, whole wheat, or sprouted grain)

Tuna (4 ounces) (canned light tuna is lower in mercury than albacore)

Turkey (4 ounces)

Turkey ham or sausage (4 ounces)

Turnip greens (unlimited)

Walnuts (¼ cup)

Watermelon (1 cup)

Whey protein (20–25 grams)

Whole grain pasta (½ cup cooked)

Yogurt, nonfat, plain, high protein preferred, Greek (½ cup)

Zucchini (unlimited)

sugar-sweetened drinks; savory snacks, such as pretzels and chips; candy; cake, pie, and pastries; fruit and fruit drinks; dairy desserts like ice cream and pudding; nuts and seeds; cookies; and milk and milk drinks.[18] Sugary, starchy, and fat-laden treats should not be your go-to snacks. Instead, focus on real food that will satisfy your hunger without undermining your weight loss program. When hunger strikes, try these sensible suggestions.

- **Nuts and seeds.** A small handful (¼ cup) of raw or dry-roasted, preferably unsalted nuts and/or seeds is one of the best snacks around. You'll fill up and get plenty of heart-healthy magnesium and vitamin E to boot. Almonds, which are rich in monounsaturated oils, top the list, but pumpkin seeds, sunflower seeds, walnuts, and most any other type of nuts are also good.

- **Edamame.** Just ½ cup of fresh soybeans provides 8 grams of protein, 5 grams of fiber, and less than 100 calories.

- **Celery with nut butter.** A stick of celery with a tablespoon or so of peanut butter combines fiber and protein for the perfect between-meals treat. Almond butter makes a nice substitution, as does a little low-fat cream cheese.

- **Cottage cheese.** Fiber-rich veggies—chopped tomatoes, bell peppers, or a little salsa—tossed in ¼ to ½ cup of low-fat or fat-free cottage cheese makes a wonderful snack. The cottage cheese provides the lean protein you need to stay satisfied, and the tasty vegetables spruce up an otherwise bland food.

- **Hard-cooked egg.** If you're looking for a low-carb, protein-rich treat, a hard-cooked egg certainly fits the bill. At just under 80 calories, this snack will curb your appetite and help trim your waistline.

- **Reduced-fat cheese.** A 1-ounce portion of reduced-fat cheese (the size of a pair of dice) has 6 to 7 grams of protein and 60 to

80 calories. String cheese is a good option, as it's easy to take with you for a snack on the run.

- **Vegetables with dip.** Cut up some fresh broccoli, carrots, tomatoes, snap peas, bell pepper strips, and/or cauliflower florets and dip them in a little hummus or light ranch dip. The calorie count of the veggies is low, plus they're full of fiber.

- **Greek yogurt.** Stir a little fruit plus stevia or xylitol as needed into ½ cup of plain nonfat Greek yogurt. Because it contains twice as much protein and half the carbohydrates of regular yogurt, it makes a terrific snack.

TO RECAP:
EAT WHAT YOU WANT

I have built this program up as a "nondiet diet," so I'm not going to pull the rug out from under you now and tell you exactly what to eat. The mini-fast with exercise accommodates a wide variety of food preferences. Michael, whom you'll read about at the end of this chapter, thrives on meat and potatoes and said up front that he couldn't abide a diet that forbade burgers and steaks. He attributes his weight loss—26 pounds and counting—in part to the fact that he isn't limited in his food selections. Hal, from Chapter 5, feels the same way about his sweets, yet he got down to his ideal weight and has stayed there.

What they and others have done, however, is to make concessions in different areas. Michael is eating smaller portions and more salads and vegetables. Hal and Lewis, discussed earlier in this chapter, both simply eat less at mealtime. If there's a particular food that you just can't do without, then by all means eat it—just have it in moderation and as part of the mini-fast with exercise.

"I FEEL SO GOOD ON THE MINI-FAST— AND IT'S SAVING MY HEALTH"

Cindy Lumpkin, from Sycamore, Illinois, was a contestant in the *Health & Healing* Diabesity Challenge. She started the mini-fast with exercise on October 10, 2010, and by November 20, she had lost 21 pounds. Then the holidays rolled around, which, as every dieter knows, can be a land mine. From Thanksgiving through Christmas, she continued to skip breakfast, but she eased up on her exercise and allowed herself the occasional sweets and larger portions that tempt us all at that time of year. During the remainder of her 12-week program, she lost only 1 more pound, ending with a total loss of 22 pounds— something anyone could be proud of.

Despite the holiday slowdown, Cindy loves the Mini-Fast Diet, and she's back on track. "I feel so good on the mini-fast—and it's saving my health! I've told so many people about it because they've noticed my weight loss."

The most important thing is to refrain from eating until noon (or several hours before and after your exercise session if you are working out later in the day). Fasting coupled with aerobic exercise transitions your body into fat burning and pushes you into ketosis. Eating shuts down this desirable function like water dousing a wildfire, and it defeats the entire purpose.

When you do break your fast, choose foods that will advance, rather than work against, your weight loss efforts. You do not have to completely give up the foods you like, even if you know they're not ideal. Just be sensible and mind your portions. If you love chocolate, have a square or two of rich dark chocolate rather than a super-size Snickers. Have a hankering for a hamburger? Hold the double meat, cheese and fries. And if you really miss breakfast, have bacon (preferably turkey) and eggs at noon. Before you know it, you will have a leaner body, a more efficient metabolism, insulin-sensitive cells, and better overall health.

Michael Carney: "Didn't Have to Give Up Meat and Potatoes"

"I have been struggling with my weight for the last 5 years or so. I'm 55 years old, and I was tipping the scales at 253 pounds. I also had high cholesterol, hypertension, and I suffered a stroke in February 2011 that caused me to lose the peripheral vision in my right eye. My health problems prompted me to visit the Whitaker Wellness Institute in March of 2011, and, boy, am I glad I went. In addition to helping me get a handle on my other conditions, my physician at the clinic started me on the mini-fast with exercise program.

"After returning home, I kept up the fasting/exercise regimen. I work out at least 3 days a week using the elliptical machine for 30 minutes, and then lifting light weights for about 15 minutes afterward. At first I thought skipping breakfast would be hard, but I find that physical activity—along with drinking lots of water and taking my supplements first thing—actually fills me up and curbs my appetite.

"My favorite part of this program is that I don't have to make major compromises when it comes to what I'm eating. Although I've adjusted my diet a little—smaller portions and more salads and vegetables—I haven't really had to change what I normally eat. This is important to me because I'm a 'meat and potatoes' kind of guy. I knew I wouldn't be able to stick with a diet that didn't allow hamburgers, steak, and the like, and I attribute my success to the fact that I don't feel restricted in my food choices.

"I've been on the mini-fast since I left the clinic, and so far I've lost 26 pounds and 2 inches from my waist. My goal is to get down to 215, so I've still got 12 pounds to go, but with this program I have no doubt that I can do it. I have more energy and I feel better than I have in a long time. I'm moving around a lot quicker these days, and this newfound vitality is really keeping me motivated."

CHAPTER 12

RECIPES

BRUNCH

SCRAMBLED EGGS WITH LOX

PREP TIME: 5 MINUTES ■ COOK TIME: 10 MINUTES
MAKES 4 SERVINGS

> 1 teaspoon olive oil
>
> 1 medium red onion, chopped
>
> 4 ounces smoked salmon, sliced into thin strips
>
> 6 large eggs
>
> 2 tablespoons low-fat milk
>
> 1 tablespoon grated Swiss cheese

1. Coat a large skillet with cooking spray and heat over medium heat. Add the olive oil and cook the onion for 1 minute. Add the salmon and cook for 2 minutes, or until the salmon begins to turn opaque and lighter in color.

2. Whisk together the eggs and milk and add to the skillet. Cook until the eggs are firm and almost dry, about 5 minutes, stirring to heat evenly.

3. Sprinkle the cheese over the eggs, and stir until melted.

Per serving: 172 calories, 16 g protein, 4 g carbohydrates, 10 g total fat, 3 g saturated fat, 1 g fiber, 335 mg sodium

BAKED HERBED EGGS

PREP TIME: 10 MINUTES ■ COOK TIME: 20 MINUTES
MAKES 2 SERVINGS

   4 eggs
   1 tablespoon all-purpose flour
   ½ teaspoon baking powder
   4 dry-packed sun-dried tomatoes, chopped
   1 tablespoon chopped fresh parsley
   1 tablespoon chopped fresh cilantro
   1 tablespoon chopped fresh dill
   2 tablespoons finely chopped red onion
   2 tablespoons chopped walnuts
   2 teaspoons finely grated lemon peel
   ¼ teaspoon salt
   ⅛ teaspoon turmeric
   ¼ teaspoon freshly ground black pepper
     Juice of ½ lemon

1. Preheat the oven to 350°F. Coat a 9" pie plate with cooking spray.
2. In a large bowl, beat the eggs, flour, and baking powder for 2 minutes. Add the sun-dried tomatoes, parsley, cilantro, dill, onion, walnuts, lemon peel, salt, turmeric, and pepper.
3. Scrape the mixture into the pie plate and bake for 20 minutes, or until lightly browned and firm to the touch. Squeeze the lemon juice over the eggs.
4. Cut into 4 wedges.

Note: Feel free to use any blend of fresh herbs or just one type if that's all you have.

Per serving: 226 calories, 15 g protein, 10 g carbohydrates, 15 g total fat, 4 g saturated fat, 1 g fiber, 639 mg sodium

TURKEY BACON AND EGG SANDWICH

PREP TIME: 5 MINUTES ■ COOK TIME: 10 MINUTES
MAKES 1 SANDWICH

1 sprouted whole grain English muffin, halved

1 slice turkey bacon

1 egg

Pinch of freshly ground black pepper

2 tablespoons shredded reduced-fat Cheddar cheese

2 slices tomato

1. Toast the English muffin halves.

2. In a small nonstick skillet over medium heat, cook the bacon for 3 minutes per side, or until crisp. Transfer to a plate lined with paper towels to drain.

3. Return the skillet to the heat. Add the egg, breaking the yolk, and sprinkle with the pepper. Cook for 1½ minutes, or until starting to set. Flip the egg over, sprinkle with the cheese, cover, and cook for 1 minute, or until the cheese melts and the egg is cooked through.

4. Place 1 muffin half on a plate. Top with the bacon, egg, tomato slices, and the other muffin half.

Per sandwich: 270 calories, 18 g protein, 18 g carbohydrates, 14 g total fat, 5 g saturated fat, 4 g fiber, 611 mg sodium

ASPARAGUS FRITTATA

PREP TIME: 5 MINUTES ■ COOK TIME: 10 MINUTES
MAKES 1 SERVING

½ tablespoon olive oil

½ cup chopped asparagus

1 small red onion, chopped

1 large egg

2 egg whites

2 tablespoons low-fat milk

1 tablespoon grated Swiss cheese

1. Preheat the broiler. Coat a small ovenproof skillet with cooking spray and heat over medium heat. Add the oil. Cook the asparagus and onion for 5 to 7 minutes, or until lightly browned.

2. Whisk together the egg, egg whites, and milk. Add to the skillet. Stir to distribute the onion and asparagus. Cook for 1 minute without stirring. Remove the skillet from the heat.

3. Sprinkle the egg mixture with the cheese. Broil for 1 to 2 minutes, or until the cheese browns and the top of the frittata is firm.

4. Cut into 4 wedges.

Per serving: 255 calories, 19 g protein, 13 g carbohydrates, 14 g total fat, 4 g saturated fat, 2 g fiber, 275 mg sodium

GOAT CHEESE SOUFFLÉS

PREP TIME: 10 MINUTES ■ COOK TIME: 30 MINUTES
MAKES 6 SERVINGS

1 tablespoon butter

2 tablespoons all-purpose flour

1 cup fat-free evaporated milk

4 eggs, separated, at room temperature

½ teaspoon cream of tartar

½ cup (4 ounces) semisoft goat cheese, crumbled

2 tablespoons chopped parsley

¼ teaspoon nutmeg

½ teaspoon salt

1. Preheat the oven to 400°F. Coat six 1-cup ramekins or baking dishes with cooking spray and place them on a baking sheet.

2. In a small saucepan over medium heat, melt the butter. Add the flour and cook, stirring, until evenly blended. Slowly whisk in the evaporated milk and bring to a simmer (the mixture will thicken quickly). Remove the white sauce from the heat and let it cool.

3. In a medium bowl, combine the egg whites and cream of tartar. Beat with an electric mixer on medium speed until frothy. Increase to high speed and beat until soft peaks form. Set aside.

4. In a separate bowl, stir together the cooled white sauce, the goat cheese, parsley, nutmeg, and salt until evenly blended. Add the egg yolks and stir well to incorporate.

5. Stir one-third of the beaten egg whites into the goat cheese mixture, gently mixing until evenly blended. Add the remaining egg whites and gently fold in, until just combined. Do not overmix.

6. Divide the soufflé mixture among the ramekins. Place the soufflés in the oven and immediately lower the oven temperature to 350°F. Bake for 25 minutes, or until puffed and slightly golden.

Per serving: 178 calories, 12 g protein, 8 g carbohydrates, 11 g total fat, 6 g saturated fat, 0 g fiber, 367 mg sodium

CHEESE GRITS WITH BACON

PREP TIME: 5 MINUTES ■ COOK TIME: 30 MINUTES
MAKES 4 SERVINGS

4 slices turkey bacon

2½ cups water

Pinch salt

½ cup grits (not instant)

½ cup grated sharp Cheddar cheese

2 scallions, coarsely chopped

1. Cook the bacon according to package directions to crisp doneness. Drain the bacon on paper towels. When cooled, crumble into bits.

2. Meanwhile, place the water in a small saucepan. Add the salt and bring to a boil. Pour the grits into the water in a thin stream, whisking to prevent clumping. Reduce the heat. Simmer the grits until fully cooked, about 12 minutes, stirring occasionally.

3. Stir in the cheese, scallions, and bacon.

Per serving: 162 calories, 10 g protein, 16 g carbohydrates, 6 g total fat, 3 g saturated fat, 1 g fiber, 132 mg sodium

BAKED CINNAMON FRENCH TOAST

PREP TIME: 10 MINUTES ■ COOK TIME: 15 MINUTES
MAKES 4 SERVINGS

2 slices sprouted wheat bread, toasted and cut into ½" cubes

4 eggs

½ cup low-fat milk

1 teaspoon vanilla extract

2 tablespoons xylitol, divided

1 cup 0% Greek yogurt

¼ teaspoon ground cinnamon

1. Preheat the oven to 350°F. Coat an 8" × 8" baking pan with cooking spray. Place the toast cubes in the pan.

2. In a medium bowl, beat the eggs, milk, vanilla, and 1 table-spoon of the xylitol with a fork. Pour over the bread. Press the bread down with a fork until soaked.

3. Bake for 15 minutes, or until puffed and set.

4. Meanwhile, in a small bowl, stir together the yogurt, cinnamon, and the remaining 1 tablespoon xylitol.

5. Cut the French toast into 4 servings. Serve with the yogurt.

Per serving: 169 calories, 13 g protein, 17 g carbohydrates, 6 g total fat, 2 g saturated fat, 1 g fiber, 174 mg sodium

BLUEBERRY PANCAKES WITH SYRUP

PREP TIME: 10 MINUTES ■ COOK TIME: 10 MINUTES
MAKES 4 SERVINGS (2 PANCAKES PER SERVING)

⅔ cup whole wheat pastry flour

⅓ cup almond flour

2 teaspoons xylitol

1¼ teaspoons baking powder

⅛ teaspoon salt

⅔ cup fat-free milk

1 egg, lightly beaten

2 teaspoons canola oil

½ teaspoon vanilla extract

½ cup blueberries

4 tablespoons blueberry fruit sweetened syrup

1. In a large bowl, combine the whole wheat flour, almond flour, xylitol, baking powder, and salt. In a separate bowl, combine the milk, egg, oil, and vanilla. Stir the milk mixture into the flour mixture until smooth. Gently fold in the blueberries.

2. Coat a large nonstick skillet with cooking spray and place over medium heat. Spoon 4 scant ¼ cupfuls of the batter into the skillet and cook for 2 to 3 minutes, or until the tops are covered with bubbles and the edges look cooked. Flip and cook for 2 minutes, or until browned on the second side. Transfer to a plate and keep warm. Repeat with the remaining batter and cooking spray as needed. Serve 2 pancakes per person, drizzled with 1 tablespoon syrup.

Per serving: 227 calories, 7 g protein, 31 g carbohydrates, 9 g total fat, 1 g saturated fat, 4 g fiber, 266 mg sodium

STRAWBERRY YOGURT FOOL

PREP TIME: 10 MINUTES ■ COOK TIME: 5 MINUTES
MAKES 1 SERVING

1 cup sliced strawberries

1 teaspoon xylitol

1 container (6 ounces) 0% Greek yogurt

2 tablespoons walnuts, toasted and chopped

In a medium bowl, mash the strawberries and xylitol. Fold in the yogurt and top with the walnuts.

Per serving: 311 calories, 19 g protein, 39 g carbohydrates, 10 g total fat, 1 g saturated fat, 4 g fiber, 100 mg sodium

CHOCO–PEANUT BUTTER SMOOTHIE

PREP TIME: 10 MINUTES ■ COOK TIME: 5 MINUTES
MAKES 1 SERVING

$\frac{1}{2}$ cup 0% Greek yogurt

$\frac{1}{2}$ cup fat-free milk

2 tablespoons natural peanut butter

2 tablespoons xylitol

2 tablespoons unsweetened cocoa powder

In a blender, combine the yogurt, milk, peanut butter, xylitol, and cocoa. Blend until smooth.

Per serving: 201 calories, 12 g protein, 27 g carbohydrates, 9 g total fat, 2 g saturated fat,
3 g fiber, 108 mg sodium

SALADS & SANDWICHES

ROASTED CORN, AVOCADO, AND BLACK BEAN SALAD

PREP TIME: 10 MINUTES ■ COOK TIME: 10 MINUTES
MAKES 4 SERVINGS

  3 tablespoons olive oil, divided
  1 cup fresh or frozen and thawed corn kernels
  1 can (15 ounces) no-salt-added black beans, rinsed and drained
  1 avocado, cubed
  2 cups cherry tomatoes, halved
  ½ small red onion, chopped
  3 tablespoons chopped fresh cilantro
  ½ teaspoon ground cumin
  2 tablespoons fresh lime juice
  1 jalapeño pepper, seeded and finely chopped (optional; wear plastic gloves when handling)
  ½ teaspoon sea salt

1. In a large nonstick skillet over medium-high heat, heat 1 tablespoon of the oil. Add the corn and cook, stirring occasionally, for 5 to 6 minutes, or until the corn starts to brown.

2. Transfer the corn to a large bowl and stir in the beans, avocado, tomatoes, onion, cilantro, cumin, lime juice, pepper, salt, and the remaining 2 tablespoons oil. Serve immediately.

Per serving: 260 calories, 6 g protein, 24 g carbohydrates, 17 g total fat, 2 g saturated fat, 8 g fiber, 242 mg sodium

ASIAN BEEF SALAD

PREP TIME: 20 MINUTES ■ COOK TIME: 20 MINUTES
MAKES 4 SERVINGS

1 teaspoon minced fresh ginger

2 tablespoons finely chopped garlic, divided

1 pound tri-tip beef

Juice of 1 lime

2 tablespoons rice vinegar

1 tablespoon fish sauce (available at Asian grocers) or less-sodium soy sauce

1 teaspoon Thai chili-garlic sauce (available at Asian grocers)

1 teaspoon toasted sesame oil

6 cups shredded Napa cabbage

4 carrots, shredded

1 red bell pepper, thinly sliced

¼ cup fresh basil leaves (Thai basil, if available), coarsely chopped

¼ cup fresh cilantro, coarsely chopped

1 small cucumber, peeled and thinly sliced

2 scallions, thinly sliced

2 tablespoons dry-roasted unsalted peanuts

1. Preheat the broiler or grill. Pat the ginger and 1 tablespoon of the garlic into the beef, coating all sides. Broil or grill the meat for 7 to 10 minutes per side, depending on thickness, or until a thermometer inserted in the center registers 145°F for medium-rare or 160°F for medium. Let sit for 10 minutes before slicing across the grain into 12 slices.

2. Meanwhile, in a small bowl, whisk together the remaining 1 tablespoon garlic, the lime juice, vinegar, fish or soy sauce, chili-garlic sauce, and sesame oil. Set the dressing aside.

3. In a large bowl, toss together the cabbage, carrots, bell pepper, basil, cilantro, cucumber, and scallions. Place the salad on a large platter.

4. Arrange the sliced meat over the salad. Drizzle with the dressing and sprinkle with the nuts.

Per serving: 298 calories, 28 g protein, 13 g carbohydrates, 15 g total fat, 4 g saturated fat, 4 g fiber, 505 mg sodium

TOSSED GREEK SALAD

PREP TIME: 20 MINUTES + CHILLING TIME
MAKES 4 SERVINGS

¾ cup whole wheat couscous

1 cup grape tomatoes, halved

1 red bell pepper, chopped

2 cucumbers, chopped

2 cups baby spinach

2 tablespoons chopped fresh parsley

2 cloves garlic, minced

½ cup crumbled reduced-fat feta cheese

¼ cup fresh lemon juice

3 tablespoons extra-virgin olive oil

¼ teaspoon salt

⅛ teaspoon freshly ground black pepper

1. Prepare the couscous according to package directions. Place in a large bowl.

2. Add the tomatoes, bell pepper, cucumbers, spinach, parsley, garlic, cheese, lemon juice, oil, salt, and black pepper to the couscous. Stir thoroughly, cover, and refrigerate until chilled, at least 1 hour and up to 1 day ahead of serving. Stir thoroughly before serving.

Per serving: 263 calories, 9 g protein, 29 g carbohydrates, 13 g total fat, 3 g saturated fat, 6 g fiber, 377 mg sodium

CUCUMBER AND RED ONION SALAD

PREP TIME: 10 MINUTES + STANDING TIME
MAKES 4 SERVINGS

- 2 large cucumbers, peeled, halved lengthwise, and thinly sliced crosswise
- 1 small red onion, thinly sliced
- 2 tablespoons rice vinegar
- 2 tablespoons chopped fresh parsley
- 2 tablespoons olive oil
- 2 teaspoons xylitol
- ¼ teaspoon salt
- ¼ teaspoon freshly ground black pepper

1. In a large bowl, combine the cucumbers and onion. In a small bowl, mix the vinegar, parsley, oil, xylitol, salt, and pepper.

2. Pour the dressing over the vegetables and toss well. Let stand for 15 minutes, tossing occasionally, before serving.

Per serving: 90 calories, 1 g protein, 7 g carbohydrates, 7 g total fat, 1 g saturated fat, 1 g fiber, 150 mg sodium

ITALIAN CHOPPED SALAD

PREP TIME: 15 MINUTES ■ MAKES 4 SERVINGS

4 cups chopped romaine lettuce

1 medium tomato, chopped

1 yellow or red bell pepper, chopped

½ small red onion, chopped

¼ cup fresh chopped basil (optional)

2 tablespoons kalamata olives, chopped

¼ cup low-fat Italian salad dressing

2 cans (5 ounces each) water-packed light tuna, drained

1 can (14–16 ounces) garbanzo beans, rinsed and drained

In a large bowl, combine the lettuce, tomato, bell pepper, onion, basil (if using), and olives. Top with salad dressing, tossing to coat. Divide among 4 plates. Top each with one-quarter of the tuna and garbanzo beans.

Per serving: 203 calories, 19 g protein, 22 g carbohydrates, 4 g total fat, 0.5 g saturated fat, 5 g fiber, 544 mg sodium

CHICKEN AND GRAPE SALAD ON SPRING GREENS

PREP TIME: 10 MINUTES ■ COOK TIME: 5 MINUTES
MAKES 6 SERVINGS

¼ cup light mayonnaise

¼ cup reduced-fat sour cream

1 teaspoon lemon juice

¼ teaspoon onion powder

¼ teaspoon garlic powder

2 cups (10½ ounces) chopped cooked chicken breast

2 ribs celery, finely chopped

1 cup red seedless grapes, halved

¼ cup almonds, toasted and chopped

12 cups mixed baby greens

1. In a medium bowl, stir together the mayonnaise, sour cream, lemon juice, onion powder, and garlic powder. Stir in the chicken, celery, grapes, and almonds.

2. Divide the greens and salad among 6 plates.

Per serving: 174 calories, 17 g protein, 10 g carbohydrates, 7 g total fat, 2 g saturated fat, 3 g fiber, 158 mg sodium

OPEN-FACED MEXICAN STUFFED-TURKEY SANDWICHES

PREP TIME: 15 MINUTES ■ COOK TIME: 25 MINUTES
MAKES 4 SERVINGS

    2 teaspoons olive oil

    1 small onion, finely chopped

    1 jalapeño pepper, seeded and finely chopped (wear plastic
      gloves when handling)

    ½ teaspoon fajita seasoning

    ½ teaspoon salt, divided

    1 clove garlic, minced

    1 cup crumbled queso blanco or reduced-fat shredded Cheddar
      cheese

    1 pound 99% lean ground turkey

    4 slices sprouted whole grain bread

    4 teaspoons picante sauce

    1 cup mixed greens

    1 tomato, cut into 4 slices

1. In a medium nonstick skillet over medium-high heat, heat the oil. Cook the onion, pepper, seasoning, and ¼ teaspoon of the salt, stirring occasionally, for 4 minutes, or until the onion starts to brown. Add the garlic and cook for 2 minutes. Remove from the heat and set aside to cool for 10 minutes. When the mixture has cooled completely, mix in the cheese.

2. Divide the turkey into 4 portions and shape each into a ball. Make a deep indentation in each with your finger and fill with one-quarter of the cheese mixture. Close the turkey around the cheese mixture and form each ball into a patty that's 3½" in diameter. Sprinkle the patties with the remaining ¼ teaspoon salt.

3. Coat a nonstick grill pan or skillet with cooking spray and heat over medium-high heat. Cook the patties for 14 to 16 minutes, turning once, until cooked through.

4. Brush each slice of bread with 1 teaspoon picante sauce. Top each with ¼ cup greens, a turkey patty, and a tomato slice. Serve.

Per serving: 328 calories, 40 g protein, 22 g carbohydrates, 10 g total fat, 3.5 g saturated fat, 4 g fiber, 622 mg sodium

GRILLED TURKEY WITH RASPBERRY DRESSING

PREP TIME: 5 MINUTES ■ COOK TIME: 10 MINUTES
MAKES 4 SERVINGS

4 teaspoons Dijon mustard

2 teaspoons light mayonnaise

3 tablespoons all-fruit raspberry spread

4 turkey breast cutlets (4 ounces each)

1 tablespoon extra-virgin olive oil

¼ teaspoon freshly ground black pepper

4 slices sprouted whole grain bread, toasted

4 large romaine leaves

4 slices reduced-fat provolone cheese

1. In a small bowl, combine the mustard, mayonnaise, and raspberry spread. Set aside. Coat a nonstick grill pan or skillet with cooking spray and heat over medium-high heat. Brush the turkey cutlets with the oil and sprinkle with the pepper. Cook the turkey for 3 to 4 minutes per side, or until well marked and cooked through. Remove from the heat.

2. Brush one side of each slice of bread with 1 generous tablespoon of raspberry dressing. Top each with a romaine leaf, a slice of cheese, and a grilled turkey cutlet. Serve open-faced.

Per serving: 344 calories, 38 g protein, 23 g carbohydrates, 11 g total fat, 4 g saturated fat, 2 g fiber, 625 mg sodium

CHICKEN QUESADILLAS

PREP TIME: 15 MINUTES ■ COOK TIME: 20 MINUTES
MAKES 4 SERVINGS

2 teaspoons canola oil

1 onion, thinly sliced

3 cloves garlic, minced

⅛ teaspoon salt

2 flour tortillas (10" diameter)

8 ounces cooked chicken breast, shredded

½ cup canned black beans, rinsed and drained

1 plum tomato, diced

¾ cup shredded reduced-fat Monterey Jack cheese

2 tablespoons chopped fresh cilantro

1. In a large nonstick skillet over medium-high heat, heat the oil. Cook the onion, garlic, and salt, stirring occasionally, for 5 minutes, or until the onion is golden.

2. Place the tortillas on a work surface. Top half of each tortilla with the onion mixture. Dividing evenly, top each with half of the chicken, beans, tomato, cheese, and cilantro. Fold the top half of each tortilla over the filling to form a semicircle.

3. Wipe the skillet and heat over medium heat. Cook the quesadillas, turning once, for 5 minutes, or until the cheese is melted and the outsides are lightly browned. Transfer to a cutting board and let cool for 2 minutes before cutting each quesadilla in half.

Per serving: 326 calories, 28 g protein, 27 g carbohydrates, 11 g total fat, 4 g saturated fat, 3 g fiber, 555 mg sodium

SPICY SHRIMP QUESADILLAS

PREP TIME: 10 MINUTES ■ COOK TIME: 20 MINUTES
MAKES 4 SERVINGS

¾ pound large shrimp, peeled and deveined

1 teaspoon olive oil

¼ teaspoon salt

½ Hass avocado, chopped

½ small red onion, chopped

½ cup reduced-fat shredded Monterey Jack or Colby cheese

1 tablespoon chopped fresh cilantro

1 jalapeño pepper, finely chopped (optional; wear plastic gloves when handling)

6 (6") sprouted wheat tortillas

1. Preheat a grill or a grill pan to medium high.

2. In a bowl, combine the shrimp, oil, and salt and toss well. Set the shrimp on a grill rack that has been coated with cooking spray. Grill for 2½ minutes per side, or until opaque and cooked through. Transfer to a cutting board. When cool enough to handle, coarsely chop and transfer to a bowl.

3. Add the avocado, onion, cheese, cilantro, and pepper to the bowl, and toss gently to combine.

4. Place 3 of the tortillas flat and divide the shrimp mixture among them. Top with the remaining 3 tortillas. Coat a large skillet with cooking spray. Heat over medium heat and carefully place one quesadilla in the skillet. Cook until the cheese is melted and the bottom is slightly browned. Carefully turn and cook until slightly browned. Remove to a plate and keep warm. Repeat with the remaining quesadillas.

5. Cut the quesadillas into quarters and serve on a platter.

Per serving: 280 calories, 23 g protein, 25 g carbohydrates, 10 g total fat, 3 g saturated fat, 4 g fiber, 495 mg sodium

ITALIAN TUNA WRAPS

PREP TIME: 15 MINUTES ■ MAKES 4 SERVINGS

   1 can (6 ounces) water-packed light tuna, drained
   1 can (15–19 ounces) small white beans, rinsed and drained
   3 tablespoons chopped fresh basil
   2 dry-pack sun-dried tomatoes, finely chopped
   3 black olives, finely chopped
   4 cherry tomatoes, chopped
   2 tablespoons red wine vinegar
   2 tablespoons olive oil
   8 large lettuce leaves, butterhead or romaine

1. In a medium bowl, combine the tuna, beans, basil, sun-dried tomatoes, olives, cherry tomatoes, vinegar, and oil.

2. Spread about ½ cup tuna mixture down the center of each lettuce leaf. Carefully roll each leaf to form a wrap. Serve.

Per serving: 161 calories, 14 g protein, 13 g carbohydrates, 8 g total fat, 1 g saturated fat, 4 g fiber, 435 mg sodium

GRILLED TWO-CHEESE ON WHOLE GRAIN BREAD

PREP TIME: 10 MINUTES ■ COOK TIME: 10 MINUTES
MAKES 1 SERVING

> 2 slices sprouted whole grain bread
> 1 teaspoon Dijon mustard
> 1 slice (1 ounce) reduced-fat Cheddar cheese
> 2 tomato slices
> 1 slice (¾ ounce) low-fat Swiss cheese

1. Spread one side of each slice of bread with the mustard. Top one slice with the Cheddar cheese, tomato, Swiss cheese, and the remaining slice of bread.

2. Coat a small nonstick skillet with cooking spray and heat over medium heat. Lightly coat the outside of the sandwich with cooking spray and add to the skillet. Cook for 4 minutes, turning once, or until the cheese has melted and the outside of the bread is golden.

Per serving: 292 calories, 20 g protein, 36 g carbohydrates, 8 g total fat, 5 g saturated fat, 6 g fiber, 752 mg sodium

SOUPS AND STEWS

CHEESY ONION SOUP

PREP TIME: 10 MINUTES ■ COOK TIME: 1 HOUR 15 MINUTES
MAKES 4 SERVINGS

    1 tablespoon olive oil
    1 teaspoon butter
    2 pounds onions, thinly sliced
    1 tablespoon xylitol
    5 cups fat-free, low-sodium vegetable broth
    1 teaspoon herbes de Provence
    2 tablespoons sherry
    ¼ teaspoon freshly ground black pepper
    4 slices (1¼ ounces each) sprouted sourdough bread, toasted
    4 slices (¾ ounce each) reduced-fat Swiss cheese

1. In a Dutch oven over medium heat, heat the oil and butter. Reduce the heat to medium low. Add the onions and xylitol and cook, stirring occasionally, for 40 to 45 minutes, or until very soft and golden.

2. Stir in the broth, herbes de Provence, sherry, and pepper. Bring to a boil over medium-high heat. Reduce to a simmer and cook, uncovered, for 30 minutes.

3. Preheat the broiler. Place the bread on a baking sheet and top each slice with 1 slice cheese. Broil for 1 minute, or until the cheese melts and browns slightly.

4. Divide the soup among 4 bowls and top each with 1 cheese toast.

Per serving: 293 calories, 13 g protein, 41 g carbohydrates, 9 g total fat, 3 g saturated fat, 5 g fiber, 445 mg sodium

TORTILLA SOUP

PREP TIME: 15 MINUTES ■ COOK TIME: 1 HOUR 5 MINUTES
MAKES 4 SERVINGS

1 tablespoon olive oil

1 small zucchini, chopped

1 small red bell pepper, chopped

2 cloves garlic, chopped

1 onion, chopped

2 cans (14.5 ounces each) Mexican-style diced tomatoes

4 cups low-sodium chicken broth

2 teaspoons chili powder or no-salt chili seasoning blend

½ teaspoon cumin

¼ teaspoon salt

1 pound boneless, skinless chicken thighs, trimmed of visible fat and cut into 1" cubes

1 chipotle pepper in adobo sauce (or to taste), finely chopped

4 corn tortillas (6" diameter)

1 Hass avocado, chopped, for garnish

¼ cup finely chopped fresh cilantro, for garnish

1 lime, cut into 8 wedges, for garnish

1. In a large pot, heat the oil over medium heat. Cook the zucchini, bell pepper, garlic, and onion until the onion is lightly browned, about 5 minutes. Add the tomatoes, broth, chili powder, cumin, and salt and cook for 10 minutes. Add the chicken cubes and bring to a boil. Reduce the heat to a simmer. Stir in the chipotle pepper and cook for 20 to 30 minutes, or until the chicken is cooked through and tender.

2. While the soup simmers, preheat the oven to 350°F. Coat the tortillas on one side with cooking spray. Sprinkle a light dusting of chili powder and cumin on each tortilla. Cut the tortillas into eighths. Place on a baking sheet and bake for 20 minutes, or until crisp.

3. Ladle the soup into 4 bowls. Top each bowl with 8 tortilla wedges, about 1 tablespoon avocado, and 1 tablespoon cilantro, if desired. Serve each with 2 lime wedges.

Per serving: 323 calories, 28 g protein, 30 g carbohydrates, 9 g total fat, 2 g saturated fat, 4 g fiber, 464 mg sodium

BEEF AND VEGETABLE SOUP

PREP TIME: 10 MINUTES ■ COOK TIME: 35 MINUTES
MAKES 6 SERVINGS

2 teaspoons olive oil

¾ pound well-trimmed beef tri-tip or bottom round, cut into
½" cubes

3 cloves garlic, minced

1 teaspoon Italian seasoning

2 cups peeled and cubed butternut squash (about 1"–2")

2 cans (14.5 ounces each) no-salt-added petite-cut diced
tomatoes

2 cups low-sodium chicken broth

1 bag (6 ounces) baby spinach

½ teaspoon salt

¼ teaspoon freshly ground black pepper

1. In a nonstick Dutch oven over medium-high heat, heat the oil.
   Cook the beef for 4 to 5 minutes, turning occasionally, or
   until browned. Add the garlic and Italian seasoning and cook
   for 1 minute, stirring occasionally. Add the squash and cook
   for 1 minute. Add the tomatoes and broth, bring to a boil,
   reduce to a simmer, cover, and cook for 20 minutes, or until
   the beef and squash are tender.

2. Stir in the spinach, cover, return to a simmer, and cook for
   5 minutes, or until the spinach is cooked. Remove from the
   heat and stir in the salt and pepper.

Per serving: 179 calories, 15 g protein, 16 g carbohydrates, 7 g total fat, 2 g saturated fat,
5 g fiber, 348 mg sodium

SIMPLE FISH CHOWDER

PREP TIME: 15 MINUTES ■ COOK TIME: 40 MINUTES
MAKES 4 SERVINGS

    5 slices turkey bacon, chopped
    2 ribs celery, chopped
    1 onion, chopped
    ½ bulb fennel, chopped
    4 cloves garlic, minced
    1 tablespoon chopped parsley
    1 can (14.5 ounces) no-salt-added diced tomatoes
    1 bottle (8 ounces) clam juice
    1 cup 2% milk
1–1¼ pounds cod fillet, cut into 1" chunks
    ¼ teaspoon freshly ground black pepper

1. In a large saucepan over medium-high heat, cook the bacon for 4 to 5 minutes, or until just starting to brown. Reduce the heat to medium and add the celery, onion, fennel, garlic, and parsley. Cook, stirring occasionally, for 6 to 7 minutes, or until the vegetables are tender-crisp.

2. Stir in the tomatoes, clam juice, and milk. Bring to a boil over medium-high heat. Reduce to a simmer, cover, and cook for 18 to 20 minutes, or until the vegetables are tender.

3. Add the cod and pepper and cook for 4 to 5 minutes, or until the cod is cooked through.

Per serving: 268 calories, 42 g protein, 15 g carbohydrates, 4 g total fat, 1 g saturated fat, 3 g fiber, 300 mg sodium

AUTUMN STEW WITH QUINOA

PREP TIME: 15 MINUTES ■ COOK TIME: 35 MINUTES
MAKES 4 SERVINGS

  1 teaspoon olive oil
  1 small onion, finely chopped
  2 cloves garlic, minced
  8 ounces mushrooms, quartered
  2½ cups peeled and cubed butternut squash
  4 cups low-sodium vegetable broth, divided
  1 tablespoon fresh lemon juice
  1 teaspoon mustard
  ¼ teaspoon dried oregano
  ¼ teaspoon salt
  ⅛ teaspoon freshly ground black pepper
  ¾ cup quinoa
  8 tablespoons shredded Parmesan

1. In a large saucepan over medium heat, heat the oil. Cook the onion, garlic, mushrooms, and squash, stirring frequently, for 5 minutes. Add ½ cup of the broth, the lemon juice, mustard, oregano, salt, and pepper. Stir to coat the vegetables. Simmer, uncovered, for 8 to 10 minutes, stirring occasionally. Increase the heat to medium high and add the remaining 3½ cups broth. Simmer for 8 to 10 minutes, or until the squash is nearly cooked through.

2. Stir in the quinoa. Cover the pan, reduce the heat to a simmer, and cook for 10 to 12 minutes, until the quinoa is tender but still a bit chewy.

3. Divide the stew among 4 bowls and garnish each portion with 2 tablespoons cheese.

Per serving: 260 calories, 12 g protein, 39 g carbohydrates, 7 g total fat, 3 g saturated fat, 6 g fiber, 511 mg sodium

DINNERS

PEACH-GLAZED PORK TENDERLOIN

PREP TIME: 15 MINUTES ■ COOK TIME: 35 MINUTES
MAKES 4 SERVINGS

1 tablespoon butter

3 cloves garlic, minced

1 small jalapeño pepper, seeded and finely chopped (wear plastic gloves when handling)

½ cup peach fruit spread

⅓ cup white wine

1 pound well-trimmed pork tenderloin

½ teaspoon salt

1. Coat a grill rack or roasting pan with cooking spray. Preheat the grill or broiler to medium high.

2. In a small saucepan over medium-high heat, melt the butter. Cook the garlic and pepper for 3 to 4 minutes, stirring, until fragrant. Add the preserves and wine, bring to a boil, and cook for 5 minutes, stirring occasionally, or until thickened slightly. Remove the saucepan from the heat. Measure out 2 tablespoons of the sauce and set aside.

3. Sprinkle the pork with the salt. Grill or broil for 15 minutes, brushing twice with the peach mixture, until a thermometer inserted into the thickest part of the tenderloin registers 160°F.

4. Transfer to a cutting board and let rest for 10 minutes before cutting into 12 slices. Top each serving with 1½ teaspoons of the reserved sauce.

Per serving: 250 calories, 24 g protein, 21 g carbohydrates, 5 g total fat, 3 g saturated fat, 0 g fiber, 373 mg sodium

GRILLED TRI-TIP WITH ESPRESSO-CHILI RUB

PREP TIME: 5 MINUTES + STANDING TIME
COOK TIME: 20 MINUTES ■ MAKES 4 SERVINGS

      2 teaspoons xylitol
      1 teaspoon instant espresso powder or fine-ground instant coffee
      ½ teaspoon mustard powder
      ½ teaspoon ground cumin
  1½ teaspoons chili powder
      1 teaspoon freshly ground black pepper
      ½ teaspoon salt
      ¼ teaspoon ground red pepper
      1 pound tri-tip steak

1. Coat a grill rack or roasting pan with cooking spray. Preheat the grill or broiler to medium high.

2. In a small bowl, combine the xylitol, espresso powder or instant coffee, mustard powder, cumin, chili powder, black pepper, salt, and red pepper. Rub all over the surface of the steak.

3. Grill or broil the steak for 4 to 6 minutes, turning once, or until a thermometer inserted in the center reads 145°F for medium-rare or 160°F for medium.

4. Let sit for 5 minutes before carving into 12 thin slices.

Per serving: 171 calories, 24 g protein, 3 g carbohydrates, 7 g total fat, 2 g saturated fat, 0 g fiber, 353 mg sodium

LONDON BROIL WITH CHIMICHURRI SAUCE

PREP TIME: 15 MINUTES ■ COOK TIME: 15 MINUTES
MAKES 4 SERVINGS

3 tablespoons chopped fresh cilantro

3 tablespoons chopped fresh parsley

2 tablespoons red wine vinegar

2 tablespoons finely chopped shallots

2 cloves garlic, peeled

¼ teaspoon crushed red pepper

2 teaspoons lime juice

1½ tablespoons extra-virgin olive oil

½ teaspoon salt, divided

¼ teaspoon freshly ground black pepper, divided

1 pound London broil or flank steak, trimmed of visible fat

1. Preheat the broiler. Coat a broiler pan with cooking spray.

2. In a food processor, combine the cilantro, parsley, vinegar, shallots, garlic, red pepper, lime juice, oil, ¼ teaspoon of the salt, and ⅛ teaspoon of the black pepper and pulse until finely chopped.

3. Sprinkle the steak with the remaining ¼ teaspoon salt and the remaining ⅛ teaspoon black pepper. Broil the steak 4" from the heat for 10 to 12 minutes, turning once, or until a thermometer inserted in the center reads 145°F for medium-rare or 160°F for medium.

4. Transfer to a cutting board and let sit for 5 minutes before cutting across the grain into 12 slices. Serve the chimichurri sauce alongside.

Per serving: 277 calories, 33 g protein, 4 g carbohydrates, 14 g total fat, 4 g saturated fat, 1 g fiber, 374 mg sodium

STEAK WITH CREAMY MADEIRA ONIONS AND MUSHROOMS

PREP TIME: 15 MINUTES ■ COOK TIME: 35 MINUTES
MAKES 4 SERVINGS

1 teaspoon olive oil

1 pound onions, thinly sliced

8 ounces baby bella mushrooms, sliced

14 ounces beef sirloin tip steak, trimmed of visible fat

½ teaspoon dried thyme

½ teaspoon dried rosemary

½ teaspoon coarse salt

½ cup fat-free, reduced-sodium beef broth

⅓ cup Madeira wine

1 tablespoon butter

2 tablespoons half-and-half

¼ teaspoon freshly ground black pepper

2 tablespoons chopped fresh parsley

1. In a large nonstick skillet coated with cooking spray, heat the oil over medium heat. Cook the onions and mushrooms for 15 minutes, stirring occasionally, or until the onions are soft and browned.

2. Coat a grill rack or roasting pan with cooking spray. Preheat the grill or broiler to medium high. Cut the steak into 4 equal pieces. Sprinkle with the thyme, rosemary, and salt.

3. Grill or broil the steak for 5 to 7 minutes, turning once, or until a thermometer inserted in the center reads 145°F for medium-rare or 160°F for medium.

4. Meanwhile, add the broth and wine to the onion mixture in the skillet and increase the heat to medium high. Cook for 4 minutes, stirring occasionally, or until the liquid has reduced by half. Add the butter and half-and-half and cook for 2 minutes, or until thickened and creamy. Season with the pepper and parsley.

5. Transfer the steaks to individual plates and spoon the onion mixture alongside.

Per serving: 294 calories, 24 g protein, 14 g carbohydrates, 14 g total fat, 6 g saturated fat, 1 g fiber, 443 mg sodium

GREEK-STYLE MEATBALLS

PREP TIME: 15 MINUTES ■ COOK TIME: 25 MINUTES
MAKES 4 SERVINGS

MEATBALLS

1 pound lean ground turkey breast

1 egg, lightly beaten

1 cup coarsely chopped spinach

2 cloves garlic, minced

1 tablespoon fresh lemon juice

1¼ teaspoons ground cumin

1¼ teaspoons dried oregano

¼ teaspoon salt

¼ teaspoon freshly ground black pepper

½ cup whole wheat panko bread crumbs

¼ cup reduced-fat feta cheese

YOGURT SAUCE

1 container (6 ounces) 0% plain Greek yogurt

1 small cucumber, peeled, seeded, and chopped

1 clove garlic, minced

2 tablespoons fresh mint

1 tablespoon lemon juice

1. Preheat the oven to 350°F. Line a baking sheet with foil and coat the foil with cooking spray.

2. *To make the meatballs:* In a medium bowl, combine the turkey, egg, spinach, garlic, lemon juice, cumin, oregano, salt, pepper, bread crumbs, and feta and mix until evenly blended. Divide the mixture in half and form each half into 8 golf ball–size meatballs.

3. Transfer the meatballs to the baking sheet and bake for 10 minutes. Turn the meatballs over and bake for 10 to 12 minutes, or until cooked through.

4. *To make the yogurt sauce:* Meanwhile, in a small bowl, combine the yogurt, cucumber, garlic, mint, and lemon juice and stir until evenly blended.

5. Serve the meatballs with the sauce alongside.

Per serving: 278 calories, 29 g protein, 12 g carbohydrates, 12 g total fat, 4 g saturated fat, 2 g fiber, 397 mg sodium

MOUSSAKA

PREP TIME: 30 MINUTES ■ COOK TIME: 1 HOUR
MAKES 6 SERVINGS

> 1 large eggplant (about 1 pound), peeled and cut crosswise into ½"-thick slices
>
> 1 tablespoon butter
>
> 3 tablespoons whole wheat panko bread crumbs
>
> 1 teaspoon olive oil
>
> 1 small onion, finely chopped
>
> 2 cloves garlic, minced
>
> 1 teaspoon cinnamon
>
> 2 teaspoons dried oregano
>
> ¾ teaspoon coarse salt, divided
>
> ¼ teaspoon freshly ground black pepper
>
> ½ pound lean ground beef
>
> ½ pound lean ground turkey breast
>
> 2 teaspoons fresh lemon juice
>
> 3 tablespoons no-salt-added tomato paste
>
> 1 can (14.5 ounces) no-salt-added petite-cut diced tomatoes, drained
>
> 1 cup low-fat (2%) evaporated milk
>
> 2 teaspoons arrowroot or cornstarch
>
> ⅓ cup reduced-fat feta cheese

1. Preheat the oven to 450°F. Line a baking sheet with foil and coat the foil with cooking spray.

2. Place the eggplant slices on the baking sheet (they can over-lap). Coat the tops with cooking spray. Bake for 18 to 20 minutes, or until lightly golden and tender. Remove from the oven and reduce the oven temperature to 350°F.

3. Meanwhile, in a medium nonstick skillet over medium heat, melt the butter. Add the bread crumbs and cook for 1 minute, stirring, or until golden. Transfer to a plate and set aside.

4. Coat the same skillet with cooking spray. Add the oil and heat over medium heat. Cook the onion, garlic, cinnamon, oregano, ½ teaspoon of the salt, and the pepper for 2 minutes, stirring, or until the onion begins to soften. Add the beef and turkey and cook for 5 minutes, breaking up the meat with a spoon, or until cooked through. Add the lemon juice, tomato paste, and tomatoes and cook, stirring, until simmering. Continue to simmer, stirring occasionally, for 5 to 7 minutes, or until the liquid is absorbed. Remove from the heat. Set aside until ready to assemble the casserole.

5. In a small saucepan, whisk together the milk, arrowroot or cornstarch, and the remaining ¼ teaspoon salt. Bring to a boil over medium-high heat, stirring constantly. When the sauce boils, it will thicken immediately. Remove from the heat and set the white sauce aside.

6. *To assemble the moussaka:* Coat an 8" × 8" baking dish with cooking spray. Make a single layer of eggplant slices in the baking dish (they can overlap), using half of the eggplant slices. Top with the meat mixture. Add a second layer of eggplant slices. Pour the white sauce over the eggplant, then sprinkle evenly with the feta cheese and the buttered bread crumbs.

7. Bake for 25 to 30 minutes, or until bubbling and golden. Let sit for 10 minutes before serving.

Per serving: 236 calories, 22 g protein, 18 g carbohydrates, 9 g total fat, 4 g saturated fat, 4 g fiber, 478 mg sodium

MOROCCAN LAMB CHOPS WITH GARBANZO RELISH

PREP TIME: 10 MINUTES ■ COOK TIME: 10 MINUTES
MAKES 4 SERVINGS

1 cup no-salt-added garbanzo beans, rinsed

1 teaspoon grated orange peel

3 tablespoons finely chopped red onion

2 tablespoons chopped fresh parsley

½ teaspoon salt, divided

¾ teaspoon ground cumin

¼ teaspoon ground cardamom

¼ teaspoon ground coriander

¼ teaspoon freshly ground black pepper

¼ teaspoon ground cinnamon

8 bone-in loin lamb chops (4 ounces each), well trimmed

1. Coat a grill rack or broiler rack with cooking spray. Preheat the grill or broiler to medium high.

2. In a small bowl, combine the garbanzo beans, orange peel, onion, parsley, and ¼ teaspoon of the salt and mix well.

3. In another small bowl, mix the cumin, cardamom, coriander, pepper, cinnamon, and the remaining ¼ teaspoon salt. Sprinkle over both sides of the lamb chops to coat.

4. Grill or broil the chops for 3½ to 4 minutes per side, or until well marked and a thermometer inserted in the center reads 145°F for medium-rare. Serve with the garbanzo relish.

Per serving: 278 calories, 32 g protein, 13 g carbohydrates, 10 g total fat, 3 g saturated fat, 3 g fiber, 388 mg sodium

OVEN-ROASTED CHICKEN BREASTS WITH BALSAMIC-GLAZED CARROTS

PREP TIME: 10 MINUTES ■ COOK TIME: 20 MINUTES
MAKES 4 SERVINGS

   3 teaspoons extra-virgin olive oil, divided

   4 boneless, skinless chicken breast halves (5–6 ounces each)

   ¼ teaspoon salt

   ¼ teaspoon freshly ground black pepper

   2 cups sliced carrots

   ½ teaspoon dried thyme

   ½ cup fat-free, reduced-sodium chicken broth

   ½ cup balsamic vinegar

   1 tablespoon xylitol

1. Preheat the oven to 350°F. Coat a baking pan with cooking spray.

2. In a large nonstick skillet over medium-high heat, heat 2 teaspoons of the oil. Sprinkle the chicken with the salt and pepper. Cook the chicken for 2 to 3 minutes per side, or until browned. Transfer to the baking pan and bake for 8 to 10 minutes, or until a thermometer inserted into the thickest portion of the breast registers 165°F and the juices run clear.

3. Meanwhile, return the skillet to the heat and add the remaining 1 teaspoon oil. Cook the carrots and thyme, stirring often, for 1 minute. Add the broth, vinegar, and xylitol. Bring to a boil and cook, stirring occasionally, for 5 to 6 minutes, or until the liquid is slightly thickened and reduced by about half. Place the chicken on a serving dish and spoon the carrots and balsamic reduction over the top.

Per serving: 255 calories, 31 g protein, 14 g carbohydrates, 7 g total fat, 1 g saturated fat, 2 g fiber, 415 mg sodium

CHICKEN PROVENÇAL

PREP TIME: 10 MINUTES ■ COOK TIME: 50 MINUTES
MAKES 4 SERVINGS

1 tablespoon olive oil

2 cloves garlic, minced

1 pound boneless, skinless chicken breasts, cut into 2" chunks

1 eggplant, peeled and cut into 2" chunks

1 cup no-salt-added canned diced tomatoes

1 cup low-sodium chicken broth

½ cup dry white wine

1½ teaspoons dried thyme

½ teaspoon salt

¼ teaspoon freshly ground black pepper

¼ cup chopped fresh parsley

1 tablespoon chopped black olives

1. In a medium saucepan over medium heat, heat the oil. Cook the garlic for 1 minute. Add the chicken, eggplant, tomatoes, broth, wine, thyme, salt, and pepper. Stir to combine. Increase the heat to medium high and bring to a boil. Reduce to a simmer and cook for 40 to 50 minutes, or until the sauce is thickened, stirring occasionally and adjusting the heat as needed to maintain a gentle simmer.

2. Stir in the parsley and olives.

Per serving: 236 calories, 27 g protein, 12 g carbohydrates, 7 g total fat, 2 g saturated fat, 5 g fiber, 472 mg sodium

SLOW-COOKER COQ AU VIN

PREP TIME: 20 MINUTES ■ COOK TIME: 4–8 HOURS
MAKES 6 SERVINGS

- 1 ounce dried porcini mushrooms or
  1 cup sliced button mushrooms
- 1 pound carrots, cut crosswise into ½" slices
- 1 onion, finely chopped
- 1 tablespoon minced garlic
- 2 slices turkey bacon, cooked and crumbled
- 1 cup chicken broth
- 2 teaspoons dried thyme
- ¼ teaspoon freshly ground black pepper
- 6 boneless, skinless chicken thighs (2 pounds total, about 5 ounces each), trimmed of visible fat
- ¾ cup dry red wine
- 1 tablespoon tomato paste

1. If using the porcini mushrooms, in a small bowl, soak the mushrooms in enough water to cover and set aside.

2. Layer the mushrooms, carrots, onion, garlic, bacon, broth, thyme, salt, and pepper in a slow cooker. Don't mix. Top with the chicken.

3. In a small bowl, combine the wine and tomato paste. Add the soaked mushrooms and the soaking liquid to the wine mixture and mix well. Pour this mixture over the chicken.

4. Cover and cook on high for 4 hours or low for 8 hours. To serve, use tongs to lift out the chicken thighs. Stir the vegetables and sauce together and spoon over each chicken thigh.

Per serving: 280 calories, 34 g protein, 14 g carbohydrates, 7 g total fat, 2 g saturated fat, 4 g fiber, 348 mg sodium

CURRIED CHICKEN WITH CAULIFLOWER AND ZUCCHINI

PREP TIME: 15 MINUTES ■ COOK TIME: 20 MINUTES
MAKES 4 SERVINGS

- 1 teaspoon canola oil
- 1 pound boneless, skinless chicken breasts, cut into ¾" pieces
- 1 onion, finely chopped
- 4 cloves garlic, minced
- 1 tablespoon grated fresh ginger
- 2 jalapeño peppers, seeded and finely chopped (optional; wear plastic gloves when handling)
- 1½ teaspoons curry powder
- ½ teaspoon ground coriander
- ½ teaspoon ground cumin
- ⅛ teaspoon ground red pepper
- ½ teaspoon coarse salt
- ¾ cup fat-free, reduced-sodium chicken broth
- 1 large head cauliflower, cut into bite-size florets (about 8½ cups)
- 2 zucchini, cut into 1" chunks
- 1 cup lite canned coconut milk
- 1 tablespoon lime juice
- 3 tablespoons finely chopped fresh cilantro

1. Coat a large saucepan with cooking spray and place over medium-high heat. Add the oil and cook the chicken, stirring, for 4 minutes, or until almost cooked through. Transfer to a plate.

2. Reduce the heat to medium and add the onion, garlic, ginger, jalapeños, curry powder, coriander, cumin, red pepper, and salt. Stir well to combine. Add the broth and cook for 3 minutes, or until the onion begins to soften.

3. Stir in the cauliflower and zucchini. Cover and cook for 8 minutes, stirring once, or until the vegetables are tender-crisp.

4. Add the coconut milk and lime juice. Return the chicken (and any accumulated juices from the plate) to the pan and stir well. Bring to a simmer and cook for 5 minutes, or until the chicken is cooked through and the sauce has reduced slightly.

5. Stir in the cilantro.

Per serving: 276 calories, 31 g protein, 20 g carbohydrates, 9 g total fat, 4 g saturated fat, 7 g fiber, 546 mg sodium

CHICKEN TACOS WITH CORN AND BLACK BEAN SALSA

PREP TIME: 10 MINUTES ■ COOK TIME: 15 MINUTES
MAKES 4 SERVINGS

½ small red onion, thinly sliced

1 jalapeño pepper, finely chopped (wear plastic gloves when handling)

1 tablespoon fresh lime juice

2 teaspoons fajita seasoning

2–3 boneless, skinless chicken breast halves (12–16 ounces total), well trimmed

8 corn tortillas (6" diameter)

1 cup shredded romaine lettuce

½ cup corn and black bean salsa

½ cup reduced-fat sour cream

1. In a small bowl, combine the onion, pepper, and lime juice. Set aside.

2. Rub the seasoning over the chicken. Coat a nonstick grill pan with cooking spray and heat over medium-high heat. Cook the chicken breasts for 6 to 7 minutes per side, or until a thermometer inserted into the thickest portion registers 165°F and the juices run clear. Transfer to a cutting board. When cool enough to handle, cut into strips.

3. Heat the tortillas according to package directions. Top each with 2 tablespoons lettuce, 3 tablespoons chicken strips, 1 tablespoon of the onion mixture, and 1 tablespoon salsa and fold in half. Serve while the tortillas are still warm, each topped with 1 tablespoon sour cream.

Per serving: 316 calories, 24 g protein, 36 g carbohydrates, 9 g total fat, 3 g saturated fat, 2 g fiber, 562 mg sodium

SPICE-RUBBED CHICKEN THIGHS

PREP TIME: 5 MINUTES ■ COOK TIME: 25 MINUTES
MAKES 4 SERVINGS

  2 teaspoons xylitol

  1 teaspoon 5-spice powder

  1 teaspoon ground coriander

  ¾ teaspoon ground cumin

  ½ teaspoon salt

  ¼ teaspoon freshly ground black pepper

  4 bone-in, skinless chicken thighs (6 ounces each), trimmed of
    visible fat

1. Coat a grill rack with cooking spray. Preheat the grill or
   broiler to medium high.

2. In a small bowl, combine the xylitol, 5-spice powder, coriander, cumin, salt, and pepper. Rub the mixture over both sides
   of the chicken thighs. Grill or broil the chicken on the rack for
   12 minutes per side, or until a thermometer inserted into the
   thickest portion registers 170°F and the juices run clear.

Per serving: 126 calories, 19 g protein, 3 g carbohydrates, 4 g total fat, 1 g saturated fat,
0 g fiber, 375 mg sodium

HOLIDAY CRANBERRY-TURKEY MEAT LOAF

PREP TIME: 20 MINUTES ■ COOK TIME: 1 HOUR 5 MINUTES
MAKES 4 SERVINGS

    1 pound lean ground turkey breast
    1 cup finely chopped onion
    1 egg
    ½ cup whole wheat panko bread crumbs
    1½ cups chopped fresh cranberries, divided
    ¼ cup tomato sauce
    ¾ teaspoon salt
    ¼ teaspoon freshly ground black pepper
    ½ teaspoon allspice
    ¼ cup water
    2 tablespoons balsamic vinegar
    1 tablespoon ketchup
    2 tablespoons xylitol

1. In a large bowl, combine the turkey, onion, egg, bread crumbs, ½ cup of the cranberries, the tomato sauce, salt, pepper, and allspice. Blend thoroughly but gently. Coat a 9" × 5" loaf pan with cooking spray and place the turkey mixture in the pan. Bake for 45 minutes, or until a thermometer inserted into the center registers 165°F and the meat is no longer pink.

2. *To make the cranberry sauce:* Meanwhile, in a small saucepan, combine the water, vinegar, ketchup, xylitol, and the remaining 1 cup cranberries. Cover and simmer over medium-low heat for 10 minutes. Let cool for 10 minutes. Transfer to a blender (or use a handheld blender right in the pan) and process to a smooth puree. Return the puree to the saucepan and simmer over medium-low heat for 10 minutes, or until the sauce thickens.

3. Cut the meat loaf into 8 slices. Place 2 slices on 4 plates and top each with 2 tablespoons of the cranberry sauce.

Per serving: 251 calories, 26 g protein, 21 g carbohydrates, 9 g total fat, 2 g saturated fat, 4 g fiber, 672 mg sodium

STUFFED SQUASH WITH TURKEY

PREP TIME: 15 MINUTES ■ COOK TIME: 1 HOUR
MAKES 4 SERVINGS

1 pound lean ground turkey breast

1 tablespoon finely chopped parsley

4 ounces shiitake mushrooms, stemmed and chopped

1 onion, chopped

2 cloves garlic, minced

2 teaspoons Italian seasoning

½ teaspoon salt

¼ teaspoon freshly ground black pepper

2 acorn squash (1 pound each), halved crosswise and seeded

1. Preheat the oven to 400°F.

2. In a bowl, combine the turkey, parsley, mushrooms, onion, garlic, seasoning, salt, and pepper and mix gently but thoroughly.

3. Pack one-quarter of the turkey mixture (about ¾ cup) in each squash half. Place the squash in a baking dish. Add 1" of water, cover with foil, and bake for 1 hour, or until the squash are tender and a thermometer inserted in the stuffing registers 165°F.

Per serving: 239 calories, 25 g protein, 22 g carbohydrates, 7 g total fat, 2 g saturated fat, 3 g fiber, 379 mg sodium

ORANGE-GLAZED CORNISH HENS

PREP TIME: 20 MINUTES ■ COOK TIME: 45 MINUTES
MAKES 4 SERVINGS

    2 Cornish hens (1.25 pounds each), rinsed and patted dry
    ½ teaspoon coarse salt
    ½ teaspoon freshly ground black pepper
    ½ teaspoon dried salt-free herb seasoning
    ½ teaspoon salt-free lemon-pepper seasoning
    1 teaspoon butter
    2 tablespoons minced garlic
    ¼ cup fresh orange juice
    2 tablespoons xylitol
    2 tablespoons fresh lemon juice
    1 teaspoon grated orange peel

1. Preheat the oven to 400°F. Coat a baking sheet with cooking spray.

2. Using a sharp, heavy knife, halve the hens lengthwise. Place them skin side up on the baking sheet. Sprinkle each half with ⅛ teaspoon salt, ⅛ teaspoon pepper, ⅛ teaspoon herb seasoning, and ⅛ teaspoon lemon-pepper seasoning. Bake for 40 to 45 minutes, or until golden and cooked through.

3. Meanwhile, in a medium nonstick skillet over medium heat, melt the butter. Cook the garlic, stirring, for 3 minutes, or until softened. Add the orange juice, xylitol, and lemon juice and whisk together until smooth and simmering. Cook for 6 to 8 minutes, or until thick and marmalade-like. Remove from the heat and stir in the peel.

4. As soon as the hens are baked, brush each half with some of the glaze. Serve with the remaining glaze spooned on top.

Per serving: 371 calories, 30 g protein, 6 g carbohydrates, 25 g total fat, 7 g saturated fat, 0 g fiber, 353 mg sodium

WASABI TUNA SALAD

PREP TIME: 20 MINUTES + MARINATING TIME
COOK TIME: 5 MINUTES ■ MAKES 4 SERVINGS

1 tablespoon less-sodium soy sauce

1 tablespoon olive oil

1 teaspoon wasabi powder

1 tablespoon rice vinegar

2 tablespoons fresh lime juice

1 tablespoon brown rice syrup

1 teaspoon toasted sesame oil

4 tuna steaks (4 ounces each), about 1" thick

4 cups spring mix or baby lettuces

1 cucumber, thinly sliced

4 scallions, thinly sliced

1 tablespoon sesame seeds, toasted

VINAIGRETTE

1 tablespoon less-sodium soy sauce

1 tablespoon rice vinegar

1 teaspoon sesame oil

2 tablespoons olive oil

½ teaspoon 5-spice powder

1. In a large bowl, combine the soy sauce, olive oil, wasabi powder, vinegar, lime juice, syrup, and sesame oil. Add the tuna steaks to the bowl. Marinate for 30 minutes in the refrigerator.

2. *To make the vinaigrette:* Meanwhile, in a small bowl, whisk the soy sauce, vinegar, sesame oil, olive oil, and 5-spice powder until thoroughly combined. Set aside.

3. Preheat the grill or a seasoned grill pan to medium high. Remove the tuna steaks from the marinade and place on the grill or grill pan. Grill the tuna for 3 minutes, flip, brush with some of the marinade, and grill for 1 minute for rare, 2 minutes for medium-rare. Transfer the tuna to a cutting board and cut into ¼"-wide strips.

4. *To assemble the salads:* Place 1 cup greens on each of 4 plates. Top each with one-quarter of the cucumber. Divide the tuna slices evenly among the plates, fanning the slices over the greens. Garnish with the scallions and sesame seeds. Serve each salad with 2 tablespoons vinaigrette.

Per serving: 297 calories, 29 g protein, 12 g carbohydrates, 15 g total fat, 3 g saturated fat, 2 g fiber, 357 mg sodium

SALMON CAKES WITH HORSERADISH CREAM

PREP TIME: 15 MINUTES ■ COOK TIME: 15 MINUTES
MAKES 4 SERVINGS

1 tablespoon + 2 teaspoons olive oil

1 cup shredded zucchini, squeezed dry

1 small onion, finely chopped

1 teaspoon minced garlic

2 tablespoons chopped parsley

2 pouches (6 ounces each) boneless pink salmon, flaked

⅔ cup oats, finely ground

2 eggs, lightly beaten

HORSERADISH CREAM SAUCE

2 tablespoons light mayonnaise

2 tablespoons light sour cream

2 teaspoons prepared horseradish

⅛ teaspoon ground red pepper

1. In a medium skillet over medium-high heat, heat 1 tablespoon oil. Cook the zucchini, onion, and garlic until softened, or 5 minutes. Remove from the heat and add the parsley, salmon, oats, and eggs. Mix well and form 8 patties.

2. *To make the sauce:* In a small bowl, combine the mayonnaise, sour cream, horseradish, and pepper and refrigerate.

3. In a large nonstick skillet over medium heat, heat 2 teaspoons oil. Add the salmon cakes and cook for 6 minutes without turning, until golden on the bottom. Turn and cook for 4 to 5 minutes, or until golden and cooked through. Serve with the sauce alongside.

Per serving: 266 calories, 21 g protein, 15 g carbohydrates, 15 g total fat, 4 g saturated fat, 2 g fiber, 538 mg sodium

CHEESY CRAB CASSEROLE

PREP TIME: 15 MINUTES ■ COOK TIME: 1 HOUR
MAKES 4 SERVINGS

1 tablespoon butter

1 onion, finely chopped

2 tablespoons chopped celery

1 cup sliced mushrooms

2 tablespoons whole wheat pastry flour

½ teaspoon freshly ground black pepper

1 cup 2% milk

½ teaspoon garlic powder

1 can (12–16 ounces) lump crabmeat, drained

1 cup frozen peas

2 tablespoons chopped fresh parsley

½ cup shredded reduced-fat Cheddar cheese

¼ cup whole wheat panko bread crumbs

1. Preheat the oven to 350°F. Coat a 2-quart round baking dish with cooking spray.

2. In a medium saucepan over medium heat, melt the butter. Cook the onion, celery, and mushrooms for 5 minutes, stirring often. Sprinkle the flour, salt, and pepper over the onion mixture and mix well. Add the milk and garlic powder. Bring to a boil, reduce to a simmer, and cook for 2 minutes to thicken. Remove from the heat and stir in the crab, peas, and parsley. Spoon into the baking dish. Sprinkle the top with the cheese and bread crumbs. Cover with foil.

3. Bake for 30 minutes, remove the foil, and bake for 15 minutes, or until browned, crisp, and bubbling.

Per serving: 271 calories, 29 g protein, 18 g carbohydrates, 9 g total fat, 4.5 g saturated fat, 3 g fiber, 487 mg sodium

PASTA PRIMAVERA WITH HALIBUT

PREP TIME: 20 MINUTES ■ COOK TIME: 25 MINUTES
MAKES 6 SERVINGS

1 pound skinless halibut fillets

1 teaspoon olive oil

2 cloves garlic, minced

1 large shallot, minced

¼ cup white wine

1½ cups low-sodium vegetable broth

¼ cup part-skim ricotta cheese

1 tablespoon fresh basil

1 tablespoon fresh thyme

¼ teaspoon sea salt

¼ teaspoon black pepper

8 ounces whole wheat penne

4 asparagus spears, cut into 1" pieces

1 cup fresh or frozen peas

¼ cup grated Parmesan cheese

1. Coat a nonstick skillet with cooking spray and heat over medium-high heat. Cook the halibut for 9 to 10 minutes, turning once, or until lightly browned and the fish flakes easily with a fork. Transfer to a plate and keep warm.

2. In a medium saucepan over medium heat, heat the oil. Cook the garlic and shallot for 5 minutes, or until golden. Add the wine and cook until almost evaporated. Add the broth, stir, and bring to a boil. Reduce the heat and simmer for 5 to 7 minutes.

3. Add some of the hot broth to the ricotta and whisk until smooth. Slowly add the ricotta to the broth in the pan and stir in the basil, thyme, salt, and pepper. Remove from the heat and set aside.

4. Bring a large pot of water to a boil. Cook the pasta according to package directions. In the last 5 minutes of cooking, add the asparagus and peas. Drain and place in a large serving bowl.

5. Gently flake the halibut into 1" chunks, add to the pasta and vegetables, and toss with the ricotta sauce. Top each serving with 2 teaspoons Parmesan.

Per serving: 310 calories, 26 g protein, 37 g carbohydrates, 6 g total fat, 2 g saturated fat, 5 g fiber, 234 mg sodium

HALIBUT WITH EASY REMOULADE SAUCE

PREP TIME: 10 MINUTES ■ COOK TIME: 10 MINUTES
MAKES 4 SERVINGS

¼ cup light mayonnaise

¼ cup chopped celery

1 tablespoon Dijon mustard

1 teaspoon prepared horseradish

1 tablespoon ketchup

1 teaspoon Worcestershire sauce

¼ teaspoon sweet paprika

4 skinless halibut fillets (4 ounces each)

¼ teaspoon salt

¼ teaspoon freshly ground black pepper

1. In a small bowl, combine the mayonnaise, celery, mustard, horseradish, ketchup, Worcestershire sauce, and paprika and mix well. Place in the refrigerator.

2. Coat a nonstick grill pan or skillet with cooking spray and heat over medium-high heat. Sprinkle the halibut with the salt and pepper and cook, turning once, for 6 minutes, or until the fish flakes easily with a fork. Remove from the heat.

3. Divide the halibut among 4 plates and serve with the sauce.

Per serving: 185 calories, 24 g protein, 4 g carbohydrates, 8 g total fat, 1 g saturated fat, 0 g fiber, 481 mg sodium

FISH TACOS WITH MANGO SALSA

PREP TIME: 15 MINUTES ■ COOK TIME: 8 MINUTES
MAKES 4 SERVINGS

    3 cups coleslaw mix
    1 teaspoon chopped jalapeño pepper (optional; wear plastic gloves when handling)
    Juice of ½ lime (about 1 tablespoon)
    ¼ cup light sour cream
    1 tablespoon xylitol
    ½ teaspoon salt, divided
    ¾ pound tilapia fillet
    4 sprouted wheat tortillas (8" diameter)

SALSA

    ¼ cup chopped fresh cilantro
    2 plum tomatoes, chopped
    1 mango, peeled and chopped
    ¼ cup chopped red onion
    Juice of 1 lime (about 2 tablespoons)

1. In a medium bowl, combine the coleslaw, pepper, lime juice, sour cream, xylitol, and ¼ teaspoon of the salt. Refrigerate.

2. *To make the salsa:* In a small bowl, mix the cilantro, tomatoes, mango, onion, and lime juice and set aside.

3. Preheat the broiler to low. Broil the tilapia about 8" from the heat for 4 minutes per side, or until cooked through. Sprinkle with remaining salt. When cool, flake the fish with a fork.

4. Warm the tortillas per package instructions.

5. Top tortillas with equal amounts of tilapia, slaw, and salsa.

Per serving: 270 calories, 23 g protein, 37 g carbohydrates, 5 g total fat, 2 g saturated fat, 5 g fiber, 460 mg sodium

SALMON PACKETS WITH BABY BOK CHOY

PREP TIME: 15 MINUTES ■ COOK TIME: 15 MINUTES
MAKES 4 SERVINGS

1 tablespoon orange peel

1 teaspoon minced ginger

3 tablespoons less-sodium soy sauce

1 tablespoon orange juice

2 teaspoons rice vinegar

2 teaspoons toasted sesame oil

4 wild salmon fillets (6 ounces each)

2 heads baby bok choy, thinly sliced

½ red bell pepper, sliced

1. Preheat the oven to 450°F. Cut 4 sheets of parchment paper into 12" × 10" rectangles. Coat each sheet with cooking spray.

2. In a small bowl, combine the orange peel, ginger, soy sauce, orange juice, and vinegar. Slowly whisk in the sesame oil.

3. Place a fillet on one-half of each sheet of parchment. Top each with one-quarter of the bok choy and bell pepper slices. Spoon the orange juice mixture over the fillets and vegetables, dividing it evenly among the packets. Fold the parchment loosely over the filling and fold the edges in to seal the packet.

4. Place the packets on a large baking sheet. Bake for 10 to 12 minutes, or until the packets are puffed. Remove from the oven and carefully vent the top of each with the tip of a sharp knife. Let sit for 1 minute. Place a packet on each of 4 serving plates, carefully fold back the parchment, and serve.

Per serving: 285 calories, 35 g protein, 4 g carbohydrates, 13 g total fat, 2 g saturated fat, 1 g fiber, 533 mg sodium

FISHERMAN'S STEW

PREP TIME: 15 MINUTES ■ COOK TIME: 6½–8½ HOURS
MAKES 4 SERVINGS

> 2 tablespoons olive oil
>
> 2 cans (14.5 ounces each) no-salt-added crushed tomatoes
>
> 1 small onion, chopped
>
> 1 cup dry white wine
>
> 1 green bell pepper, chopped
>
> 1 jalapeño pepper, chopped (optional; wear plastic gloves when handling)
>
> 1 teaspoon dried thyme
>
> 2 teaspoons dried basil
>
> 1 teaspoon dried oregano
>
> 1 quart low-sodium chicken broth
>
> ½ pound cod fillet
>
> ½ pound peeled and deveined shrimp, tails removed
>
> ½ pound sea scallops

1. In a large skillet, heat the oil over medium-high heat. Cook the tomatoes and onion for 5 minutes, or until the onion is softened. Add the wine and simmer for 10 minutes. Add the bell pepper, jalapeño pepper, thyme, basil, and oregano. Place the contents of the skillet in a 4- to 6-quart slow cooker, add the broth, and cook on low for 6 to 8 hours.

2. Turn the slow cooker to high and add the cod, shrimp, and scallops. Cook for 15 to 30 minutes, or until the seafood is cooked through.

Per serving: 292 calories, 27 g protein, 23 g carbohydrates, 8 g total fat, 1 g saturated fat, 5 g fiber, 616 mg sodium

OVEN-FRIED CATFISH
WITH CAJUN TARTAR SAUCE

PREP TIME: 15 MINUTES ■ COOK TIME: 15 MINUTES
MAKES 4 SERVINGS

3 tablespoons yellow mustard

2 tablespoons red wine vinegar

½ teaspoon crushed red-pepper flakes

Pinch of salt

2 egg whites, lightly beaten

¼ cup cornmeal

¼ cup whole wheat panko bread crumbs

½ teaspoon onion powder

¼ teaspoon garlic powder

4 catfish fillets (4 ounces each)

½ teaspoon freshly ground black pepper

TARTAR SAUCE

⅓ cup 0% plain Greek yogurt

1 tablespoon pickle relish

1 tablespoon light mayonnaise

¼ teaspoon ground cumin

¼ teaspoon paprika

1. Preheat the oven to 450°F. Coat a baking sheet with cooking spray.

2. In a shallow bowl, combine the mustard, vinegar, pepper flakes, and salt. Place the egg whites in a second shallow bowl. In a third shallow bowl, combine the cornmeal, bread crumbs, onion powder, and garlic powder. Sprinkle the catfish with the pepper and salt to taste. Working with one fillet at a time, dredge both sides of the fillet in the mustard mixture. Dip the fillet in the egg whites and then in the cornmeal mixture. Place each fillet on the baking sheet.

3. *To make the tartar sauce:* In a bowl, mix together the yogurt, pickle relish, mayonnaise, cumin, and paprika and set aside.

4. Lightly coat the fillets with cooking spray and bake for 7 minutes. Turn the fillets over, coat with cooking spray, and bake for 5 to 6 minutes, or until the fish is cooked through and crisp. Top with the tartar sauce and serve.

Per serving: 242 calories, 23 g protein, 13 g carbohydrates, 11 g total fat, 2.5 g saturated fat, 2 g fiber, 327 mg sodium

MARYLAND CRAB CAKES WITH REMOULADE SAUCE

PREP TIME: 20 MINUTES ■ COOK TIME: 20 MINUTES
MAKES 4 SERVINGS

2 tablespoons chopped parsley

1 egg + 2 egg whites, beaten

3 tablespoons light mayonnaise

1 teaspoon dry mustard

2 teaspoons fresh lemon juice

½ small onion, chopped

½ teaspoon hot sauce

1 pound lump crabmeat

½ cup whole wheat panko bread crumbs

REMOULADE SAUCE

3 tablespoons light mayonnaise

¼ teaspoon celery salt

2 tablespoons finely chopped celery

2 tablespoons finely chopped red onion

1 teaspoon prepared horseradish

1. *To make the crab cakes:* In a large bowl, combine the parsley, egg and egg whites, mayonnaise, mustard, lemon juice, onion, and hot sauce and mix well. Stir in the crabmeat. Add the bread crumbs and mix gently until just combined.

2. Divide the crab cake mixture into 12 even portions (¼ cup each) and form into ½" cakes.

3. Coat a large nonstick skillet with cooking spray and heat over medium heat. Add 6 crab cakes to the pan. Coat the top of each crab cake with cooking spray and cook for 3 to 5 minutes, or until the crab cakes are golden on the bottom.

4. Flip the crab cakes and cook for 3 to 5 minutes, or until cooked through. Transfer to a plate and cover with foil to keep warm. Repeat with the remaining crab cakes.

5. *To make the sauce:* Combine the mayonnaise, celery salt, celery, onion, and horseradish. Serve the crab cakes with the sauce.

Per serving: 277 calories, 32 g protein, 11 g carbohydrates, 10 g total fat, 2 g saturated fat, 2 g fiber, 707 mg sodium

SHRIMP SCAMPI WITH QUINOA

PREP TIME: 10 MINUTES ■ COOK TIME: 20 MINUTES
MAKES 4 SERVINGS

1 cup quinoa

1 tablespoon olive oil

5 cloves garlic, minced

½ teaspoon sea salt

¼ teaspoon freshly ground black pepper

Pinch of red-pepper flakes

¼ cup dry white wine

½ cup reduced-sodium chicken broth

1 teaspoon grated lemon peel

1 pound peeled and deveined large shrimp, tails removed

¼ cup finely chopped fresh flat-leaf parsley

1. Cook the quinoa according to package directions and set aside.

2. In a large nonstick skillet over medium heat, heat the oil. Cook the garlic, salt, black pepper, and pepper flakes for 3 minutes, stirring, or until the garlic is softened. Add the wine and broth. Increase the heat and bring to a simmer. Cook for 2 minutes to slightly reduce the liquid.

3. Add the lemon peel and shrimp. Cook for 4 minutes, stirring once or twice, or until the shrimp are opaque and cooked through. Pour the shrimp mixture over the quinoa. Add small amounts of broth to thin the sauce, if needed. Garnish with the parsley and serve.

Per serving: 309 calories, 27 g protein, 31 g carbohydrates, 8 g total fat, 1 g saturated fat, 3 g fiber, 510 mg sodium

MARGARITA MUSHROOM PIZZA

PREP TIME: 10 MINUTES ■ COOK TIME: 30 MINUTES
MAKES 8 SERVINGS

1 tablespoon extra-virgin olive oil

8 ounces mushrooms, sliced

1 onion, chopped

1 teaspoon dried oregano

¼ teaspoon salt

¼ teaspoon freshly ground black pepper

4 cloves garlic, minced

1 sprouted or whole grain pizza shell (16 ounces) (see note)

2 plum tomatoes, cut into 12 slices total

½ cup shredded part-skim mozzarella cheese

⅓ cup grated Parmesan cheese

¼ cup fresh basil leaves

1. Preheat the oven to 400°F. Coat a baking sheet with cooking spray.

2. In a large nonstick skillet over medium-high heat, heat the oil. Cook the mushrooms, onion, oregano, salt, and pepper, stirring occasionally, for 9 to 10 minutes. Add the garlic and cook for 3 minutes, or until browned. Remove from the heat.

3. Place the pizza shell on the baking sheet. Arrange the tomato slices over the shell in a single layer. Top with the mushroom mixture, mozzarella, Parmesan, and basil. Bake for 17 to 20 minutes, or until the crust is crisp and the cheese is melted and lightly browned. Remove from the oven and let cool briefly before cutting into 8 slices.

Note: Look for these products in the frozen section of the natural foods section of your market.

Per serving: 257 calories, 10 g protein, 38 g carbohydrates, 7 g total fat, 2 g saturated fat, 2 g fiber, 381 mg sodium

SPINACH-STUFFED EGGPLANT ROLLATINI

PREP TIME: 30 MINUTES ■ COOK TIME: 40 MINUTES
MAKES 6 SERVINGS

2 large eggplants

1 package (10 ounces) frozen chopped spinach, thawed and squeezed dry

1 container (15 ounces) part-skim ricotta cheese

1 egg

2 tablespoons grated Parmesan cheese

1 tablespoon Italian seasoning

¼ teaspoon garlic powder

1 tablespoon olive oil

½ onion, chopped

2 cloves garlic, minced

1 can (28 ounces) crushed tomatoes with Italian seasonings

½ cup water

1 cup shredded part-skim mozzarella cheese

¼ cup chopped fresh parsley

1. Preheat the broiler. Coat a 3"-deep 3-quart baking dish with cooking spray.

2. Cut the tips off the eggplants. Slice each eggplant lengthwise into six ¼" slices. Coat the eggplant slices with cooking spray and broil on a baking sheet for 15 minutes, or until golden brown. Remove from the oven and cool.

3. Meanwhile, in a medium bowl, combine the spinach, ricotta, egg, Parmesan, Italian seasoning, and garlic powder and blend well.

4. In a medium saucepan over medium heat, heat the oil. Cook the onion and garlic, stirring occasionally, for 4 to 5 minutes, or until the onion has softened and is starting to brown. Stir in the tomatoes and water. Bring the mixture to a low boil, reduce to a simmer, and cook for 5 minutes. Keep the tomato sauce warm while you roll up the eggplant.

5. Working with one slice at a time, place the eggplant slices on a cutting board. Using a small spatula, scoop ¼ cup of the spinach-ricotta mixture onto the eggplant and spread it evenly. Roll up the eggplant, patting in any filling that starts to squeeze out. Place the roll on its side (not end up) in the baking dish. Repeat with the remaining eggplant slices and the remaining spinach-ricotta filling.

6. Pour the tomato sauce over the roll-ups. Cover the baking dish with a lid or foil. Bake for 15 minutes, or until the sauce is bubbling. Remove from the oven, uncover, and sprinkle with the mozzarella. Bake for 5 minutes, or until the cheese is melted. Let stand for 5 minutes. Sprinkle with the parsley before serving.

Per serving: 305 calories, 21 g protein, 25 g carbohydrates, 14 g total fat, 7 g saturated fat, 9 g fiber, 623 mg sodium

CUBAN-STYLE QUINOA AND BEANS

PREP TIME: 10 MINUTES ■ COOK TIME: 40 MINUTES
MAKES 4 SERVINGS

4 teaspoons extra-virgin olive oil

1 onion, chopped

1 large red bell pepper, chopped

3 cloves garlic, minced

1 teaspoon dried basil

1 teaspoon ground cumin

½ teaspoon ground coriander

2 teaspoons Creole seasoning

Dash of ground red pepper

16 grape or cherry tomatoes

¼ cup apple cider vinegar

2 cans (15 ounces each) no-salt-added black beans, rinsed and drained

½ teaspoon salt

¼ teaspoon freshly ground black pepper

¾ cup quinoa

1. In a large saucepan over medium-high heat, heat the oil. Cook the onion, bell pepper, garlic, basil, cumin, coriander, seasoning, and red pepper, stirring occasionally, for 5 minutes.

2. Add the tomatoes and cook for 3 minutes. Add the vinegar and cook for 30 seconds. Add the beans, bring to a boil, reduce to a simmer, cover, and cook for 30 minutes, stirring occasionally, or until the vegetables are very tender. Season with the salt and pepper.

3. Meanwhile, cook the quinoa according to package directions and top with the bean mixture.

Per serving: 326 calories, 14 g protein, 50 g carbohydrates, 8 g total fat, 1 g saturated fat, 11 g fiber, 616 mg sodium

SOUTHWEST PORTOBELLO STACK

PREP TIME: 15 MINUTES ■ COOK TIME: 15 MINUTES
MAKES 4 SERVINGS

    2 cloves garlic, minced
½–2 teaspoons hot-pepper sauce
    1 tablespoon olive oil
    1 teaspoon Worcestershire sauce
    2 tablespoons balsamic vinegar
    4 portobello mushrooms (4 ounces each), stems removed
    ¼ teaspoon salt
    ⅛ teaspoon freshly ground black pepper
    ½ cup shredded pepper Jack cheese
    1 tomato, cut into 4 thick slices
    2 sprouted whole grain burger buns, halved
    1 avocado, pitted and sliced
    4 thin slices red onion (from ½ small)

1. Preheat the grill to medium high or the broiler to high. Coat a grill rack or broiler pan with cooking spray.

2. In a small bowl, combine the garlic, hot sauce, oil, Worcestershire sauce, and balsamic vinegar. Brush the mushrooms with the vinegar mixture and sprinkle with the salt and pepper.

3. Set the mushrooms gill side down on the grill rack or broiler pan. Grill or broil for 6 minutes, or until they begin to soften. Turn and top with the cheese. Grill or broil for 6 to 7 minutes, or until tender. Meanwhile, coat the tomato slices with cooking spray and grill or broil for 1 minute on each side.

4. Set one-half of each bun on 4 plates. Top each with a portobello, a tomato slice, one-quarter of the avocado, and an onion slice.

Per serving: 282 calories, 11 g protein, 27 g carbohydrates, 16 g total fat, 4 g saturated fat, 7 g fiber, 411 mg sodium

SAVORY BEAN PATTIES WITH TAHINI SAUCE

PREP TIME: 35 MINUTES + REFRIGERATION TIME ■ COOK TIME: 15 MINUTES
MAKES 4 SERVINGS

GARBANZO PATTIES

1½ teaspoons olive oil

4 scallions, chopped

2 cloves garlic, finely chopped

2 tablespoons dried porcini mushroom slices

2 cans (15 ounces each) garbanzo beans, rinsed and drained

¼ cup sprouted whole wheat bread crumbs (about ½ slice)

1 egg

1 tablespoon dried oregano

1½ teaspoons ground cumin

½ teaspoon salt

½ teaspoon freshly ground black pepper

TAHINI SAUCE

½ cup low-fat plain yogurt

2 tablespoons tahini

1 tablespoon lemon juice

⅓ cup fresh flat-leaf parsley, chopped

4 cups mixed greens

1 cucumber, thinly sliced

1. *To make the patties:* In a large skillet over medium heat, heat the oil. Cook the scallions and garlic for 2 minutes, or until the scallions are softened. Remove from the heat.

2. Process the mushroom slices in a food processor until finely chopped. Add the garbanzo beans and process until just finely chopped; do not puree. Transfer to a large mixing bowl. Add the scallion mixture, the bread crumbs, egg, oregano, cumin, salt, and pepper. Mix well. Refrigerate for at least 15 minutes or up to 1 hour.

3. Form the bean mixture into 8 small patties. Coat a large skillet with olive oil cooking spray and place over medium heat. Cook the patties (in 2 batches, if necessary) for 3 minutes, or until lightly browned and crisp on the bottom. Turn them over, gently press down with a spatula to flatten them slightly, and cook for 3 minutes, or until lightly browned and crisp on the other side.

4. *To make the sauce:* In a small bowl, combine the yogurt, tahini, lemon juice, and parsley.

5. Assemble 2 patties over 1 cup mixed greens and top with the cucumber slices. Drizzle with the tahini sauce and serve.

Per serving: 264 calories, 13 g protein, 34 g carbohydrates, 10 g total fat, 2 g saturated fat, 8 g fiber, 655 mg sodium

ASIAN GRILLED TOFU STEAKS OVER NAPA SLAW

PREP TIME: 15 MINUTES + MARINATING TIME
COOK TIME: 10 MINUTES ■ MAKES 4 SERVINGS

1 package (14 ounces) extra-firm tofu

4 tablespoons rice vinegar, divided

2 cloves garlic, minced

2 tablespoons minced ginger

1 tablespoon less-sodium soy sauce

1 Napa cabbage, shredded

1 package (8 ounces) sliced cremini or brown mushrooms

3 tablespoons chopped scallions

1 teaspoon sesame oil

1 tablespoon extra-virgin olive oil

1 teaspoon Dijon mustard

1 teaspoon xylitol

½ teaspoon salt

¼ teaspoon freshly ground black pepper

1. Place the tofu on a stack of several paper towels and for about 1 minute gently press out excess moisture. Cut lengthwise into 4 thin slices.

2. In a shallow glass or ceramic dish (that will hold the tofu snug in one layer), combine 2 tablespoons of the vinegar, the garlic, ginger, and soy sauce. Add the tofu slices, turning to coat. Marinate at room temperature for 30 minutes.

3. In a large bowl, combine the cabbage and mushrooms. In a small bowl, mix the scallions, sesame oil, olive oil, mustard, xylitol, salt, pepper, and the remaining 2 tablespoons vinegar. Pour the scallion mixture over the cabbage mixture and toss well. Divide among 4 plates.

4. Coat a nonstick grill pan with cooking spray and heat over medium-high heat. Remove the tofu from the marinade and add to the grill pan. Grill the tofu for 3 minutes per side, or until well marked and hot. Serve the grilled tofu over the Napa slaw.

Per serving: 208 calories, 15 g protein, 17 g carbohydrates, 10 g total fat, 1 g saturated fat, 4 g fiber, 501 mg sodium

DESSERTS

CHOCOLATE-ALMOND BISCOTTI

PREP TIME: 30 MINUTES ■ COOK TIME: 45 MINUTES
MAKES 10 SERVINGS (2 BISCOTTI PER SERVING)

¾ cup whole wheat pastry flour

¼ cup unsweetened cocoa powder

¾ teaspoon baking soda

¼ teaspoon sea salt

⅔ cup xylitol or xylitol brown sweetener

2 eggs

1 tablespoon brewed coffee

½ teaspoon vanilla extract

¼ cup chopped almonds

⅓ cup bittersweet chocolate chips

1. Preheat the oven to 350°F. Line a baking sheet with parchment paper.

2. In a medium bowl, whisk together the flour, cocoa, baking soda, salt, and xylitol.

3. In a small bowl, lightly beat the eggs. Reserve 1 tablespoon of the beaten egg and set aside in a separate bowl. Whisk the coffee and vanilla into the remaining eggs. Add the egg mixture to the flour mixture and mix with a wooden spoon until blended, about 2 minutes. The dough should be somewhat stiff and sticky.

4. On the baking sheet, shape the dough into a single log (12" long × 4" wide × 1" high). Gently press the almonds into the top of the dough. Brush the reserved 1 tablespoon egg over the top and sides of the log. Bake for 30 minutes, or until the dough is firm to the touch. Remove the cookie log and let cool for 15 minutes. Reduce the heat to 300°F.

5. Transfer the cooled cookie log to a cutting board. Using a sharp serrated knife, cut the log crosswise into 20 biscotti, about ½" wide. Place the cookies on the baking sheet (it's okay if they're touching). Bake for 12 to 15 minutes, or until crisp. Let the cookies cool completely.

6. In a microwaveable bowl, microwave the chocolate chips on high power for 1 minute and then at 12-second intervals, stirring in between, until smooth and fully melted. Dip a fork into the melted chocolate and drizzle it over the biscotti. (You may have to reheat the chocolate if it thickens too much to drizzle.) Let the biscotti sit until the chocolate cools and hardens, then store in an airtight container.

Per serving: 103 calories, 4 g protein, 17 g carbohydrates, 5 g total fat, 2 g saturated fat, 2 g fiber, 148 mg sodium

WHOOPIE PIES

PREP TIME: 45 MINUTES ■ COOK TIME: 10 MINUTES
MAKES 12 SERVINGS

>   3 tablespoons butter, at room temperature
>   ¼ cup xylitol or xylitol brown sweetener
>   1 egg white
>   ⅓ cup low-fat buttermilk
>   ½ teaspoon instant coffee granules or espresso powder
>   ½ teaspoon vanilla extract
>   ¾ cup whole wheat pastry flour
>   3 tablespoons unsweetened cocoa powder
>   1 teaspoon baking soda
>   12 tablespoons light whipped cream topping

1. Preheat the oven to 350°F. Line 2 baking sheets with parchment paper and coat the paper with cooking spray.

2. In a medium bowl, combine the butter and xylitol. Beat with an electric mixer on medium high until blended, 2 minutes. Add the egg white and beat until incorporated.

3. In a measuring cup, combine the buttermilk, coffee granules or espresso powder, and vanilla. In a small bowl, mix the flour, cocoa, and baking soda.

4. Add one-half of the flour mixture to the butter-egg mixture and beat well. Beat in one-half of the buttermilk. Repeat.

5. Scoop the batter by rounded tablespoonfuls onto the baking sheets, making 24 round portions. Bake for 10 minutes. Cool for 15 minutes.

6. To serve, squirt 1 tablespoon whipped cream onto the flat side of one cake, then top with another cake to make a sandwich. Repeat with the remaining cakes.

Per serving: 69 calories, 2 g protein, 9 g carbohydrates, 4 g total fat, 2.5 g saturated fat, 1 g fiber, 145 mg sodium

TROPICAL BLONDIES

PREP TIME: 45 MINUTES ■ COOK TIME: 30 MINUTES
MAKES 9 SERVINGS

½ cup whole wheat pastry flour

½ cup almond flour or almond meal

1¼ teaspoons baking powder

⅛ teaspoon salt

¼ cup unrefined coconut oil, melted

2 eggs

1 cup xylitol or xylitol brown sweetener

1 teaspoon coconut extract

½ teaspoon vanilla extract

⅔ cup unsweetened coconut

¼ cup finely chopped almonds

1. Preheat the oven to 350°F. Coat an 8" × 8" baking pan with cooking spray and dust lightly with flour.

2. In a small bowl, combine the whole wheat flour, almond flour or almond meal, baking powder, and salt. In a large bowl, mix the coconut oil, eggs, xylitol, coconut extract, and vanilla. Stir the flour mixture into the egg mixture until well combined. Stir in the unsweetened coconut. Pour into the baking pan. Sprinkle the top with the chopped almonds.

3. Bake for 25 to 30 minutes, or until a toothpick inserted in the center comes out with a few moist crumbs. Cool in the pan on a rack for 30 minutes. Cut into 9 bars.

Per serving: 184 calories, 4 g protein, 16 g carbohydrates, 16 g total fat, 9 g saturated fat, 3 g fiber, 120 mg sodium

RASPBERRY CHEESECAKES

PREP TIME: 1 HOUR 45 MINUTES ■ COOK TIME: 25 MINUTES
MAKES 6 SERVINGS

    2 tablespoons finely chopped pecans
    8 ounces Neufchâtel or light cream cheese, at room temperature
    ¼ cup xylitol
    ¼ teaspoon vanilla extract
    1 egg
    2 tablespoons reduced-sugar red raspberry jam or seedless
      preserves
    6 fresh raspberries

1. Preheat the oven to 350°F. Line 6 cups of a muffin pan with foil cupcake liners.

2. Place 1 teaspoon of the pecans in each cupcake liner.

3. In a medium bowl, combine the cheese, xylitol, vanilla, and egg. Using an electric mixer, beat until smooth, about 2 minutes. Divide the batter evenly among the cupcake liners, being careful not to disturb the pecans.

4. Bake for 25 minutes or until a toothpick inserted comes out clean. Let cool in the pan for 30 minutes. Refrigerate for at least 1 hour, or until chilled.

5. Just before serving, remove the cheesecakes from the liners (peel carefully) and place them on dessert plates. In a small bowl or cup, stir the jam or preserves until smooth, adding a little water if needed. Drizzle about 1 teaspoon over each cheesecake. Top each with 1 raspberry.

Per serving: 158 calories, 5 g protein, 14 g carbohydrates, 11 g total fat, 5 g saturated fat, 0 g fiber, 138 mg sodium

RUSTIC PEACH AND ALMOND CRISP

PREP TIME: 10 MINUTES ■ COOK TIME: 45 MINUTES
MAKES 8 SERVINGS

1½ pounds peaches, peeled and sliced

½ cup xylitol

1 tablespoon cornstarch

1 teaspoon ground cinnamon

¼ teaspoon ground nutmeg

¼ teaspoon almond extract

¾ cup rolled oats

¾ cup sliced almonds

2 tablespoons butter

1. Preheat the oven to 400°F. Coat an 8" × 8" baking dish with cooking spray.

2. In a large bowl, combine the peaches, xylitol, cornstarch, cinnamon, nutmeg, and almond extract and toss well. Pour into the baking dish and spread evenly.

3. In a small bowl, combine the oats and almonds. Using a fork, incorporate the butter into the oat-almond mixture. Dot the top of the peaches with the oat mixture.

4. Cover the dish tightly with foil. Bake for 30 minutes. Remove the foil and bake for 15 minutes. Serve warm.

Per serving: 245 calories, 5 g protein, 43 g carbohydrates, 11 g total fat, 3 g saturated fat, 5 g fiber, 1 mg sodium

PEANUT BUTTER COOKIES

PREP TIME: 25 MINUTES ■ COOK TIME: 35 MINUTES
MAKES 2½ DOZEN COOKIES

½ cup creamy natural peanut butter

¼ cup butter

2 eggs

½ cup xylitol

1 teaspoon vanilla extract

¾ cup whole wheat pastry flour

½ cup quinoa flour

¾ teaspoon baking soda

½ teaspoon baking powder

¼ teaspoon salt

1. In a large bowl, combine the peanut butter, butter, eggs, xylitol, and vanilla. With a hand mixer on low speed, beat until well blended, about 2 minutes.

2. In another bowl, mix the whole wheat flour, quinoa flour, baking soda, baking powder, and salt. Add the flour mixture to the peanut butter mixture and blend until the flour is incorporated to form a dough. Refrigerate for 15 minutes.

3. Preheat the oven to 375°F. Coat a baking sheet with cooking spray.

4. Shape the dough into 1¼" balls and place about 3" apart on the baking sheet. Flatten with a fork, making a crisscross pattern.

5. Bake for 10 to 12 minutes, or until golden brown.

Per cookie: 72 calories, 2 g protein, 8 g carbohydrates, 4 g total fat, 2 g saturated fat, 1 g fiber, 84 mg sodium

BROWNIES

PREP TIME: 25 MINUTES ■ COOK TIME: 45 MINUTES
MAKES 9 SERVINGS

½ cup semisweet chocolate chips

3 tablespoons butter

3 eggs

⅔ cup xylitol

1 teaspoon vanilla extract

¾ cup whole wheat pastry flour

¼ cup unsweetened cocoa powder

¾ teaspoon baking powder

⅛ teaspoon salt

1 tablespoon powdered xylitol

1. Preheat the oven to 325°F. Coat an 8" × 8" baking pan with cooking spray and line with waxed or parchment paper.

2. In a small glass bowl, combine the chocolate chips and butter. Microwave on high for 1 minute or until melted, stirring after 30 seconds.

3. In a medium bowl, whisk together the eggs, xylitol, and vanilla. Whisk in the chocolate mixture, flour, cocoa, baking powder, and salt until smooth. Pour the batter into the pan.

4. Bake for 30 to 40 minutes, or until a toothpick inserted into the center comes out nearly clean. Let cool in the pan for 10 minutes, then remove from the pan and let cool completely on a rack. Cut into 9 bars and sprinkle with the powdered xylitol before serving.

Per serving: 204 calories, 4 g protein, 34 g carbohydrates, 8 g total fat, 5 g saturated fat, 1 g fiber, 97 mg sodium

The Mini-Fast Diet 2-Week Meal Plan

Noon Meal

Blueberry Pancakes with Syrup (page 266)

2 slices turkey bacon

Snack

3 ribs celery

1½ tablespoons peanut butter

Dinner

4 ounces salmon fillet brushed with 1 teaspoon olive oil, sprinkled with salt-free lemon-pepper seasoning, and broiled

Lettuce and tomato salad

2 cups broccoli florets sautéed in 1 tablespoon olive oil with 1 clove chopped garlic

Snack

1 apple

¼ cup 0% Greek yogurt, sweetened with 1 teaspoon low-sugar jam

Noon Meal

Open-Faced Chicken Sandwich prepared with:

   1 slice sprouted grain bread

   1 teaspoon light mayonnaise

   3½ ounces cooked chicken breast

   2 slices roasted red pepper

   1 slice part-skim mozzarella cheese

Orange

Snack

¼ cup dry-roasted almonds

Dinner

Asian Grilled Tofu Steaks over Napa Slaw (page 332)

½ cup cooked soba noodles

Tossed green salad

Snack

Banana drizzled with 1 tablespoon melted dark chocolate

DAY 3

Noon Meal

Southwest Shrimp Salad prepared with:

4 ounces cooked shrimp

2 cups chopped romaine

¼ cup chopped avocado

¼ cup corn kernels

¼ cup cooked black beans

Sliced red onion, red bell pepper, and tomato

Low-fat cilantro-lime dressing

Snack

¼ cup fat-free cottage cheese

½ cup cherry tomatoes

Dinner

Steak with Creamy Madeira Onions and Mushrooms (page 292)

¾ cup cooked sweet potato

Tossed salad with julienne carrots

Snack

Strawberry Yogurt Fool (page 267)

DAY 4

Noon Meal

Savory Bean Patties with Tahini Sauce (page 330)

Pear

Snack

¼ cup steamed edamame drizzled with 1 teaspoon less-sodium soy sauce

Dinner

4 ounces roasted pork tenderloin

½ cup cooked whole wheat orzo

Steamed asparagus drizzled with lemon juice

Spinach salad

Snack

½ meal-replacement bar containing 7 grams protein and 5 grams carbohydrates

DAY 5

Noon Meal

Mango-Curry Chicken Salad Wrap. In a large bowl, combine:

1 tablespoon light mayonnaise

1 tablespoon mango chutney

¼ teaspoon curry powder

Toss in:

3½ ounces shredded cooked chicken

¼ cup chopped apple

¼ cup chopped celery

Serve in sprouted grain tortilla wrap.

Snack

1 reduced-fat string cheese stick with baby carrots

Dinner

London Broil with Chimichurri Sauce (page 291)

½ cup cooked quinoa

½ cup sautéed diced zucchini and yellow squash

Snack

1 Whoopie Pie (page 336)

DAY 6

Noon Meal

Chicken-Vegetable Soup prepared with:

   2 cups low-sodium chicken broth

   4 ounces shredded cooked chicken

   ½ cup sliced carrots

   1 cup baby spinach

Serve with ½ sprouted grain English muffin.

Snack

4 ribs celery

3 tablespoons light cream cheese

Dinner

Moroccan Lamb Chops with Garbanzo Relish (page 298)

½ cup steamed brown rice

Steamed cauliflower

Snack

½ cup sliced peaches topped with ¼ cup chopped nuts and a dollop of 0% Greek yogurt

DAY 7

Noon Meal

Southwest Burger prepared with:

   4 ounces turkey or beef burger

   1 thin slice Monterey Jack cheese

   ½ cup sautéed mushrooms

   1 tablespoon low-sodium ketchup

   1 sprouted wheat bun

Serve with cucumber slices.

Snack

1 deviled egg with bell pepper rings

Dinner

Stuffed Squash with Turkey (page 308)

Tossed green salad

Snack

1 Raspberry Cheesecake (page 338)

DAY 8

Noon Meal

Turkey Bacon and Egg Sandwich (page 260)

Snack

3 ribs celery

1½ tablespoons almond butter

Dinner

Pasta with Meat Sauce prepared with:

> 4 ounces ground beef sautéed with 1 cup sliced cherry tomatoes and 1 teaspoon dried basil, served over ½ cup cooked sprouted grain pasta, and topped with 1 tablespoon Parmesan cheese

Lettuce, tomato, and cucumber salad

Snack

Banana drizzled with 2 tablespoons semisweet chocolate chips, melted, and rolled in chopped nuts

DAY 9

Noon Meal

Open-Faced Mexican Stuffed-Turkey Sandwich (page 276)

Carrot sticks

Snack

¼ cup sunflower seeds

Dinner

4 ounces sea scallops seared in 1 tablespoon olive oil

½ cup cooked quinoa

1 cup steamed spinach

Snack

1 Tropical Blondie (page 337)

DAY 10

Noon Meal

Greek salad prepared with:

2 cups romaine

Cherry tomatoes

Sliced red onion

Kalamata olives

¼ cup crumbled reduced-fat feta cheese

Snack

¼ cup raw walnuts

Dinner

Grilled Tri-Tip with Espresso-Chili Rub (page 290)

½ baked potato topped with ¼ cup shredded reduced-fat Cheddar cheese

Grilled zucchini brushed with 1 teaspoon olive oil

Snack

½ meal-replacement bar containing 7 grams protein and 5 grams carbohydrates

DAY 11

Noon Meal

Tortilla Soup (page 284)

Snack

¼ cup steamed edamame drizzled with 1 teaspoon less-sodium soy sauce

Dinner

Asian Stir-Fry prepared with:

4 ounces diced chicken (or cubed tofu)

1 bell pepper

1 tablespoon olive oil

1 tablespoon stir-fry sauce

½ cup brown rice

Steamed spinach

Snack

Pear

1 reduced-fat string cheese stick

DAY 12

Noon Meal

Open-Faced Chicken, Brie, and Cranberry Sandwich prepared with:

1 slice sprouted grain bread

2 teaspoons all-fruit cranberry (or raspberry) spread

4 ounces cooked chicken

1 ounce sliced Brie cheese, broiled until melted

Snack

4 ribs celery

3 tablespoons light cream cheese

Dinner

Peach-Glazed Pork Tenderloin (page 289)

½ roasted acorn squash

1 cup sautéed green beans

Snack

¼ cup 0% Greek yogurt

½ cup blueberries

DAY 13

Noon Meal

Salmon Salad prepared with light mayonnaise and pickle relish

Snack

¼ cup dry-roasted almonds

Dinner

Pasta Primavera with Halibut (page 314)

Tossed salad with garbanzo beans and carrot and tomato slices

Snack

½ meal-replacement bar containing 7 grams protein and 5 grams carbohydrates

DAY 14

Noon Meal

Simple Fish Chowder (page 287)

Apple

Snack

3 cups air-popped popcorn

Dinner

Grilled Steak Tacos prepared with:

4 ounces thinly sliced grilled flank steak

2 tablespoons chopped tomatoes

2 tablespoons shredded reduced-fat cheese

1 tablespoon 0% Greek yogurt

1 sprouted wheat tortilla (6" diameter)

½ cup refried beans

Salsa

Snack

Strawberry Yogurt Fool (page 267)

Endnotes

Chapter 1

1   Jacqueline D. Wright et al., "Trends in Intake of Energy and Macronutrients—United States, 1971–2000," *Morbidity and Mortality Weekly Report* 53, no. 4 (2004): 80–2.

2   Jacqueline D. Wright and Chia-Yih Wang, *Trends in Intake of Energy and Macronutrients in Adults from 1999–2000 through 2007–2008*, NCHS Data Brief, no. 49 (Hyattsville, MD: National Center for Health Statistics, 2010).

3   Ock K. Chun et al., "Changes in Intakes of Total and Added Sugar and Their Contribution to Energy Intake in the U.S.," *Nutrients* 2, no. 8 (2010): 834–54.

4   US weight loss market forecasted to hit $66 billion in 2013. PRWeb. 2011 December 31, www.prweb.com/releases/2012/12/prweb10278281.htm.

5   Helen Truby et al., "Randomised Controlled Trial of Four Commercial Weight Loss Programmes in the UK: Initial Findings from the BBC 'Diet Trials,'" *British Medical Journal* 332, no. 7553 (2006): 1309–14.

6   Gary D. Foster et al., "Weight and Metabolic Outcomes After 2 Years on a Low-Carbohydrate versus Low-Fat Diet," *Annals of Internal Medicine* 153, no. 3 (2010): 147–57.

7   Traci Mann et al., "Medicare's Search for Effective Obesity Treatments: Diets Are Not the Answer," *American Psychologist* 62, no. 3 (2007): 220–33.

8   "NWCR Facts," National Weight Control Registry, accessed June 4, 2011, www.nwcr.ws /Research/default.htm.

9   Gary Taubes, "The Scientist and the Stairmaster," *New York*, September 24, 2007.

Chapter 2

1   Susan T. Stewart, David M. Cutler, and Allison B. Rosen, "Forecasting the Effects of Obesity and Smoking on U.S. Life Expectancy," *New England Journal of Medicine* 361 (2009): 2252–60.

2   Cynthia L. Ogden and Margaret D. Carroll, *Prevalence of Overweight, Obesity, and Extreme Obesity among Adults: United States, Trends 1960–1962 through 2007–2008*, Health E-Stats (Hyattsville, MD: National Center for Health Statistics, June 2010), www.cdc.gov/NCHS/data /hestat/obesity_adult_07_08/obesity_adult_07_08.pdf.

3   Roland Sturm, "Increases in Morbid Obesity in the USA: 2000–2005," *Public Health* 121, no. 7 (2007): 492–96.

4   Donald F. Behan and Samuel H. Cox, *Obesity and Its Relation to Mortality and Morbidity Costs* (Schaumburg, IL: Society of Actuaries, December 2010), www.soa.org/files/pdf /research-2011-obesity-relation-mortality.pdf.

5   John Cawley and Chad Meyerhoefer, *The Medical Care Costs of Obesity: An Instrumental Variables Approach*, NBER Working Paper, no. 16467 (Cambridge, MA: National Bureau of Economic Research, October 2010), www.nber.org/papers/w16467.pdf.

6   Martin A. Makary et al., "Medication Utilization and Annual Health Care Costs in Patients with Type 2 Diabetes Mellitus Before and After Bariatric Surgery," *Archives of Surgery* 145, no. 8 (2010): 726–31.

7   John D. Scott et al., "Does Bariatric Surgery Reduce the Risk of Major Cardiovascular Events? A Retrospective Cohort Study of Morbidly Obese Surgical Patients," Surgery for Obesity and Related Diseases, published electronically September 19, 2011, doi:10.1016 /j.soard.2011.09.002.

8   Teri L. Hernandez et al., "Fat Redistribution Following Suction Lipectomy: Defense of Body Fat and Patterns of Restoration," *Obesity* 19, no. 7 (2011): 1388–95.

9   John P. H. Wilding, "The Importance of Free Fatty Acids in the Development of Type 2 Diabetes," *Diabetic Medicine* 24, no. 9 (2007): 934–45.

10 Tomoaki Morioka et al., "Disruption of Leptin Receptor Expression in the Pancreas Directly Affects Beta Cell Growth and Function in Mice," *Journal of Clinical Investigation* 117, no. 10 (2007): 2860–2868.

11 Pauline Koh-Banerjee et al., "Changes in Body Weight and Body Fat Distribution as Risk Factors for Clinical Diabetes in US Men," *American Journal of Epidemiology* 159, no. 12 (2004): 1150–1159.

12 A. Singhal, "Endothelial Dysfunction: Role in Obesity-Related Disorders and the Early Origins of CVD," *Proceedings of the Nutrition Society* 64, no. 1 (2005): 15–22.

13 Isle L. Mertens and Luc F. Van Gaal, "Overweight, Obesity, and Blood Pressure: The Effects of Modest Weight Reduction," *Obesity Research* 2000, no. 8: 270–278.

14 Alan J. Flint et al., "Excess Weight and the Risk of Incident Coronary Heart Disease among Men and Women," *Obesity* 18, no. 2 (2010): 377–83.

15 Eugenia E. Calle et al., "Overweight, Obesity, and Mortality from Cancer in a Prospectively Studied Cohort of U.S. Adults," *New England Journal of Medicine* 348, no. 17 (2003): 1625–38.

16 S. A. Harrison et al., "Orlistat for Overweight Subjects with Nonalcoholic Steatohepatitis: A Randomized, Prospective Trial," *Hepatology* 49, no. 1 (2009): 80–86.

17 Ichiro Yoshikawa et al., "Long-Term Treatment with Proton Pump Inhibitor Is Associated with Undesired Weight Gain," *World Journal of Gastroenterology: WJG* 15, no. 38 (2009): 4794–98.

18 Y. J. Cheng et al., "Prevalence of Doctor-Diagnosed Arthritis and Arthritis-Attributable Activity Limitation—United States, 2007–2009," *MMWR Morbidity and Mortality Weekly Report* 59, no. 39 (2010): 1261–65.

Chapter 3

1   Babak Bahadori et al., "A 'Mini-Fast with Exercise' Protocol for Fat Loss," *Medical Hypotheses* 73, no. 4 (2009): 619–22.

2   Katherine M. Flegal et al., "Comparisons of Percentage Body Fat, Body Mass Index, Waist Circumference, and Waist-Stature Ratio in Adults," *American Journal of Clinical Nutrition* 89, no. 2 (2009): 500–508.

3   Jacqueline D. Wright and Chia-Yih Wang, *Trends in Intake of Energy and Macronutrients in Adults from 1999–2000 through 2007–2008*, NCHS Data Brief, no. 49 (Hyattsville, MD: National Center for Health Statistics, 2010).

4   Alan C. Goldhamer et al., "Medically Supervised Water-Only Fasting in the Treatment of Borderline Hypertension," *Journal of Alternative and Complementary Medicine* 8, no. 5 (2002): 643–50.

5   M. F. McCarty, "A Preliminary Fast May Potentiate Response to a Subsequent Low-Salt, Low-Fat Vegan Diet in the Management of Hypertension—Fasting as a Strategy for Breaking Metabolic Vicious Cycles," *Medical Hypotheses* 60, no. 5 (2003): 624–33.

6   Ibid.

7   John K. Davidson, *Clinical Diabetes Mellitus: A Problem-Oriented Approach*, 3rd ed. (New York: Thieme, 2000).

8   Douglas J. Lisle and Alan Goldhamer, *The Pleasure Trap* (Summertown, TN: Healthy Living Publications, 2003).

9   J. Galgani and E. Ravussin, "Energy Metabolism, Fuel Selection and Body Weight Regulation," *International Journal of Obesity* 32, Supplement 7 (2008): S109–19.

10 M. F. McCarty, "Optimizing Exercise for Fat Loss," *Medical Hypotheses* 44, no. 5 (1995): 325-30.

11 Karen Van Proeyen et al., "Training in the Fasted State Improves Glucose Tolerance during Fat-Rich Diet," *Journal of Physiology* 588 (2010): 4289–302.

12 Anthony E. Civitarese et al. "Calorie Restriction Increases Muscle Mitochondrial Biogenesis in Healthy Humans," *PLoS Medicine* 4, no. 3 (2007): e76, doi:10.1371/journal.pmed.0040076.

13 Babak Bahadori et al., "A 'Mini-Fast with Exercise' Protocol for Fat Loss," *Medical Hypotheses* 73, no. 4 (2009): 619–22.

Chapter 4

1 Kellogg Company, "Kellogg Reveals Results of Monumental Breakfast Survey," news release, June 22, 2011, http://kelloggs.mediaroom.com/index.php?s=43&item=346.

2 Volker Schusdziarra et al., "Impact of Breakfast on Daily Energy Intake—An Analysis of Absolute versus Relative Breakfast Calories," *Nutrition Journal* 10 (January 2011): 5, doi:10.1186/1475-2891-10-5.

3 Andreas von Budnoff, "The Breakfast Hype," *Los Angeles Times*, September 18, 2006, http://articles.latimes.com/2006/sep/18/health/he-breakfast18.

4 Gary Langer, "Poll: What Americans Eat for Breakfast," ABC News, *Good Morning America*, May 17, 2005, www.abcnews.go.com/GMA/PollVault/story?id=762685.

5 "Basal Energy Expenditure: Harris-Benedict Equation," Cornell University, accessed March 10, 2012, http://www-users.med.cornell.edu/~spon/picu/calc/beecalc.htm.

6 Mark P. Mattson, "The Need for Controlled Studies of the Effects of Meal Frequency on Health," *Lancet* 365, no. 9475 (2005): 1978–80.

7 Marion Nestle, *What to Eat* (New York: North Point Press, 2006).

Chapter 5

1 Daniel G. Carey, "Quantifying Differences in the 'Fat Burning' Zone and the Aerobic Zone: Implications for Training," *Journal of Strength and Conditioning Research* 23, no. 7 (2009): 2090–95.

2 L. M. Burke, "Caffeine and Sports Performance," *Applied Physiology, Nutrition, and Metabolism* 33, no. 6 (2008): 1319–34.

3 L. Wang et al., "Alcohol Consumption, Weight Gain, and Risk of Becoming Overweight in Middle-Aged and Older Women," *Archives of Internal Medicine* 170, no. 5 (2010): 453–61.

4 M. F. McCarty, "Hepatothermic Therapy of Obesity: Rationale and an Inventory of Resources," *Medical Hypotheses* 57, no. 3 (2001): 324–36.

5 Kiwon Lim et al., "(-)-Hydroxycitrate Ingestion and Endurance Exercise Performance," *Journal of Nutritional Science and Vitaminology* 51, no. 1 (2005): 1–7.

6 H. G. Preuss et al., "Effects of a Natural Extract of (-)-Hydroxycitric Acid (HCA-SX) and a Combination of HCA-SX plus Niacin-Bound Chromium and *Gymnema sylvestre* Extract on Weight Loss," *Diabetes, Obesity and Metabolism* 6, no. 3 (2004): 171–80.

7 Igho Onakpoya et al., "The Use of *Garcinia* Extract (Hydroxycitric Acid) as a Weight Loss Supplement: A Systematic Review and Meta-Analysis of Randomised Clinical Trials," *Journal of Obesity* 2011: 509038, doi:10.1155/2011/509038.

8 Nicolo Longo, Cristina Amat Di San Filippo, and Marzia Pasquali, "Disorders of Carnitine Transport and the Carnitine Cycle," *American Journal of Medical Genetics: Part C, Seminars in Medical Genetics* 142C, no. 2 (2006): 77–85.

9 Stephen D. Anton et al., "Effects of Chromium Picolinate on Food Intake and Satiety," *Diabetes Technology and Therapeutics* 10, no. 5 (2008): 405–12.

10 Max H. Pittler and Edzard Ernst, "Dietary Supplements for Body-Weight Reduction: A Systematic Review," *American Journal of Clinical Nutrition* 79, no. 4 (2004): 529–36.

11 M. F. McCarty and J. C. Gustin, "Pyruvate and Hydroxycitrate/Carnitine May Synergize to Promote Reverse Electron Transport in Hepatocyte Mitochondria, Effectively 'Uncoupling' the Oxidation of Fatty Acids," *Medical Hypotheses* 52, no. 5 (1999): 407–16.

12 Tia M. Rains, Sanjiv Agarwal, and Kevin C. Maki, "Antiobesity Effects of Green Tea Catechins: A Mechanistic Review," *Journal of Nutritional Biochemistry* 22, no. 1 (2011): 1–7.

13 Francisco Di Pierro et al., "GreenSelect Phytosome as an Adjunct to a Low-Calorie Diet for Treatment of Obesity: A Clinical Trial," *Alternative Medicine Review: A Journal of Clinical Therapeutics* 14, no. 2 (2009): 154–60.

14 Muhammad Shoaib Akhtar et al., "Effect of Amla Fruit (*Emblica officinalis* Gaertn.) on Blood Glucose and Lipid Profile of Normal Subjects and Type 2 Diabetic Patients," *International Journal of Food Sciences and Nutrition* 62, no. 6 (2011): 609–16.

15 Rebecca Kuriyan et al., "Effect of Supplementation of *Coccinia cordifolia* Extract on Newly Detected Diabetic Patients," *Diabetes Care* 31, no. 2 (2008): 216–20.

16 A. Ascherio et al., "A Prospective Study of Nutritional Factors and Hypertension among US Men," *Circulation* 86, no. 5: 1475–84.

17 S. Devaraj et al., "Low Vitamin D Levels in Northern American Adults with the Metabolic Syndrome," *Hormone and Metabolic Research* 43, no. 1 (2011): 72–74.

Chapter 6

1 Marketdata Enterprises, "Diet Market Worth $60.9 Billion in the U.S. Last Year, but Growth Is Flat, Due to the Recession," news release, May 5, 2011, www.marketdataenterprises.com /pressreleases/DietMarket2011PR.pdf.

2 Igho Onakpoya et al., "The Use of *Garcinia* Extract (Hydroxycitric Acid) as a Weight Loss Supplement: A Systematic Review and Meta-Analysis of Randomised Clinical Trials," *Journal of Obesity* 2011: 509038, doi:10.1155/2011/509038.

3 M. F. McCarty, "Hepatothermic Therapy of Obesity: Rationale and an Inventory of Resources," *Medical Hypotheses* 57, no. 3 (2001): 324–36.

4 Francisco Di Pierro et al., "GreenSelect Phytosome as an Adjunct to a Low-Calorie Diet for Treatment of Obesity: A Clinical Trial," *Alternative Medicine Review: A Journal of Clinical Therapeutics* 14, no. 2 (2009): 154–60.

5 M. Rondanelli et al., "Satiety and Amino-Acid Profile in Overweight Women after a New Treatment Using a Natural Plant Extract Sublingual Spray Formulation," *International Journal of Obesity* 33, no. 10 (2009): 1174–82.

6 A. A. Noorbala et al., "Hydro-Alcoholic Extract of *Crocus sativus* L. versus Fluoxetine in the Treatment of Mild to Moderate Depression: A Double-Blind, Randomized Pilot Trial," *Journal of Ethnopharmacology* 97, no. 2 (2005): 281–84.

7 Nicholas A. Christakis and James H. Fowler, "The Spread of Obesity in a Large Social Network over 32 Years," *New England Journal of Medicine* 357, no. 4 (2007): 370–79.

8 Ibid.

9 A. A. Gorin et al., "Weight Loss Treatment Influences Untreated Spouses and the Home Environment: Evidence of a Ripple Effect," *International Journal of Obesity* 32, no. 11 (2008): 1678–84.

Chapter 7

1 Jennifer A. Linde et al., "Self-Weighing in Weight Gain Prevention and Weight Loss Trials," *Annals of Behavioral Medicine* 30, no. 3 (2005): 210–216.

2 Jeffrey J. VanWormer et al., "Self-Weighing Frequency Is Associated with Weight Gain Prevention over 2 Years among Working Adults," *International Journal of Behavioral Medicine*, published electronically July 6, 2011, doi:10.1007/s12529-011-9178-1.

3 Jacob C. Seidell et al., "Waist and Hip Circumferences Have Independent and Opposite Effects on Cardiovascular Disease Risk Factors: The Quebec Family Study," *American Journal of Clinical Nutrition* 74, no. 3 (2001): 315–21.

4   Susan M. Majka, Yaacov Barak, and Dwight J. Klemm, "Concise Review: Adipocyte Origins: Weighing the Possibilities," *Stem Cells* 29, no. 7 (2011): 1034–40.

5   "Classification of Overweight and Obesity by BMI, Waist Circumference, and Associated Disease Risks," National Heart Lung and Blood Institute, accessed March 11, 2012, www.nhlbi.nih.gov/health/public/heart/obesity/lose_wt/bmi_dis.htm.

6   International Diabetes Federation, *The IDF Consensus Worldwide Definition of the Metabolic Syndrome* (Brussels: International Diabetes Federation, 2006), www.idf.org/webdata/docs /IDF_Meta_def_final.pdf. 2006.

7   Eric J. Jacobs et al., "Waist Circumference and All-Cause Mortality in a Large US Cohort," *Archives of Internal Medicine* 170, no. 15 (2010): 1293–301.

8   Preethi Srikanthan, Teresa E. Seeman, and Arun S. Karlamangla, "Waist-Hip-Ratio as a Predictor of All-Cause Mortality in High-Functioning Older Adults," *Annals of Epidemiology* 19, no. 10 (2009): 724–31.

9   "Body Fat Scales: Will They Help?" *Consumer Reports* 69, no. 1 (2004): 24–5.

10 Katherine M. Flegal et al., "Comparisons of Percentage Body Fat, Body Mass Index, Waist Circumference, and Waist-Stature Ratio in Adults," *American Journal of Clinical Nutrition* 89, no. 2 (2009): 500–508.

Chapter 8

1   Brian Kim, "Thyroid Hormone as a Determinant of Energy Expenditure and the Basal Metabolic Rate," *Thyroid* 18, no. 2 (2008): 141–44.

2   Zeev Arinzon et al., "Evaluation Response and Effectiveness of Thyroid Hormone Replacement Treatment on Lipid Profile and Function in Elderly Patients with Subclinical Hypothyroidism," *Archives of Gerontology and Geriatrics* 44, no. 1 (2007): 13–9.

3   Konstantinos A. Toulis et al., "Selenium Supplementation in the Treatment of Hashimoto's Thyroiditis: A Systematic Review and a Meta-Analysis," *Thyroid* 20, no. 10 (2010): 1163–73.

4   Benjamin C. Blount et al., "Urinary Perchlorate and Thyroid Hormone Levels in Adolescent and Adult Men and Women Living in the United States," *Environmental Health Perspectives* 114, no. 12 (2006): 1865–71.

5   James E. Haddow et al., "Maternal Thyroid Deficiency during Pregnancy and Subsequent Neuropsychological Development of the Child," *New England Journal of Medicine* 341, no. 8 (1999): 549–55.

6   Kent Holtorf, "The Bioidentical Hormone Debate: Are Bioidentical Hormones (Estradiol, Estriol, and Progesterone) Safer or More Efficacious Than Commonly Used Synthetic Versions in Hormone Replacement Therapy?" *Postgraduate Medicine* 121, no. 1 (2009): 73–85.

7   G. Corona, "Hypogonadism and Metabolic Syndrome," *Journal of Endocrinological Investigation* 34 (2011): 557–67.

8   Dennis T. Villareal and John O. Holloszy, "Effect of DHEA on Abdominal Fat and Insulin Action in Elderly Women and Men," *Journal of the American Medical Association* 292, no. 18 (2004): 2243–48.

9   M. Rondanelli et al., "Satiety and Amino-Acid Profile in Overweight Women after a New Treatment Using a Natural Plant Extract Sublingual Spray Formulation," *International Journal of Obesity* 33, no. 10 (2009): 1174–82.

10 Shahin Akhondzadeh et al., "Comparison of *Crocus sativus* L. and Imipramine in the Treatment of Mild to Moderate Depression: A Pilot Double-Blind Randomized Trial," *BMC Complementary and Alternative Medicine* 4 (2004): 12.

11 A. A. Noorbala et al., "Hydro-Alcoholic Extract of *Crocus sativus* L. versus Fluoxetine in the Treatment of Mild to Moderate Depression: A Double-Blind, Randomized Pilot Trial," *Journal of Ethnopharmacology* 97, no. 2 (2005): 281–84.

12 Bernard Gout, Cédric Bourges, and Séverine Paineau-Dubreuil, "Satiereal, a *Crocus sativus*

L Extract, Reduces Snacking and Increases Satiety in a Randomized Placebo-Controlled Study of Mildly Overweight, Healthy Women," *Nutrition Research* 30, no. 5 (2010): 305–13.

13 Tanja C. Adam and Elissa S. Epel, "Stress, Eating and the Reward System," *Physiology and Behavior* 91, no. 4 (2007): 449–58.

14 Jayanthi Kandiah et al., "Stress Influences Appetite and Comfort Food Preferences in College Women," *Nutrition Research* 26, no. 3 (2006): 118–23.

15 Angelika Lettner and Michael Roden, "Ectopic Fat and Insulin Resistance," *Current Diabetes Reports* 8, no. 3 (2008): 185–91.

16 *American Heritage Medical Dictionary*, s.v. "iatrogenic" (Boston: Houghton Mifflin, 2007), medical-dictionary.thefreedictionary.com/iatrogenic.

17 W. S. Leslie, C. R. Hankey, and M. E. J. Lean, "Weight Gain As an Adverse Effect of Some Commonly Prescribed Drugs: A Systematic Review," *QJM: Monthly Journal of the Association of Physicians* 100, no. 7 (2007): 395–404.

18 Christoph U. Correll et al., "Cardiometabolic Risk of Second-Generation Antipsychotic Medications during First-Time Use in Children and Adolescents," *Journal of the American Medical Association* 302, no. 16 (2009): 1765–73.

19 Francesco P. Cappuccio et al., "Meta-Analysis of Short Sleep Duration and Obesity in Children and Adults," *Sleep* 31, no. 5 (2008): 619–26.

20 Karen Spruyt, Dennis L. Molfese, and David Gozal, "Sleep Duration, Sleep Regularity, Body Weight, and Metabolic Homeostasis in School-Aged Children," *Pediatrics* 127, no. 2 (2011): e345–52.

21 Russel J. Reiter et al., "Obesity and Metabolic Syndrome: Association with Chronodisruption, Sleep Deprivation, and Melatonin Suppression," *Annals of Medicine*, published electronically June 13, 2011, doi:10.3109/07853890.2011.586365.

22 Kimberly L. Jackson, "National Sleep Awareness Week: Cell Phones, Laptops, iPads and Other Devices Are Keeping Us Up at Night," March 10, 2011, NJ.com, www.nj.com/homegarden /index.ssf/2011/03/national_sleep_awareness_week.html.

23 Jennifer Glass et al., "Sedative Hypnotics in Older People with Insomnia: Meta-Analysis of Risks and Benefits," *BMJ: British Medical Journal* 331, no. 7526 (2005): 1169.

24 Samir Malhotra, Girish Sawhney, and Promila Pandhi, "The Therapeutic Potential of Melatonin: A Review of the Science," *MedGenMed: Medscape General Medicine* 6, no. 2 (2004): 46.

25 Susan Hadley and Judith J. Petry, "Valerian," *American Family Physician* 67, no. 8 (2003): 1755–58.

26 Russ Mason, "200 mg of Zen: L-Theanine Boosts Alpha Waves, Promotes Alert Relaxation," *Alternative and Complementary Therapies* 7 (2001): 91–95.

Chapter 9

1 "NWCR Facts," National Weight Control Registry, accessed June 4, 2011, www.nwcr.ws /Research/default.htm.

Chapter 10

1 National Center for Health Statistics, *Health, United States, 2010: With Special Feature on Death and Dying* (Hyattsville, MD: National Center for Health Statistics, 2011).

2 Janet E. Fulton et al., "Physical Activity Levels of High School Students—United States, 2010," *Morbidity and Mortality Weekly Report* 60, no. 23 (2011): 773–77.

3 Nancy D. Brener et al., "Beverage Consumption among High School Students—United States, 2010," *Morbidity and Mortality Weekly Report* 60, no. 23 (2011): 778–80.

4 Emmanuel Stamatakis, Mark Hamer, and David W. Dunstan, "Screen-Based Entertainment Time, All-Cause Mortality, and Cardiovascular Events: Population-Based Study with Ongoing

Mortality and Hospital Events Follow-Up," *Journal of the American College of Cardiology* 57, no. 3 (2011): 292–99.

5 L. Alford, "What Men Should Know about the Impact of Physical Activity on Their Health," *International Journal of Clinical Practice* 64, no. 13 (2010): 1731–34.

6 Gary Taubes, "The Scientist and the Stairmaster," *New York*, September 24, 2007.

7 M. F. McCarty, "Optimizing Exercise for Fat Loss," *Medical Hypotheses* 44, no. 5 (1995): 325–30.

8 Juul Achten and Asker E. Jeukendrup, "Optimizing Fat Oxidation through Exercise and Diet," *Nutrition* 20, no. 7–8 (2004): 716–27.

9 Daniel G. Carey, "Quantifying Differences in the 'Fat Burning' Zone and the Aerobic Zone: Implications for Training," *Journal of Strength and Conditioning Research* 23, no. 7 (2009): 2090–95.

10 Fabien Pillard, "Lipid Oxidation According to Intensity and Exercise Duration in Overweight Men and Women," *Obesity* 15, no. 9 (2007): 2256–62.

11 David R. Bassett et al., "Pedometer-Measured Physical Activity and Health Behaviors in U.S. Adults," *Medicine and Science in Sports and Exercise* 42, no. 10 (2010): 1819–25.

12 Dena M. Bravata et al., "Using Pedometers to Increase Physical Activity and Improve Health: A Systematic Review," *Journal of the American Medical Association* 298, no. 19 (2007): 2296–304.

13 Simon J. Marshall et al., "Translating Physical Activity Recommendations into a Pedometer-Based Step Goal: 3,000 Steps in 30 Minutes," *American Journal of Preventive Medicine* 36, no. 5 (2009): 410–15.

14 Benoit Capostagno and Andrew Bosch, "Higher Fat Oxidation in Running Than Cycling at the Same Exercise Intensities," *International Journal of Sport Nutrition and Exercise Metabolism* 20, no. 1 (2010): 44–55.

15 Erica R. Goldstein et al., "International Society of Sports Nutrition Position Stand: Caffeine and Performance," *Journal of the International Society of Sports Nutrition* 7, no. 1 (2010): 5.

16 M. F. McCarty, "Hepatothermic Therapy of Obesity: Rationale and an Inventory of Resources," *Medical Hypotheses* 57, no. 3 (2001): 324–36.

17 Darcye J. Cuff et al., "Effective Exercise Modality to Reduce Insulin Resistance in Women with Type 2 Diabetes," *Diabetes Care* 26, no. 11): 2977–82.

18 Kevin R. Vincent and Randy W. Braith, "Resistance Exercise and Bone Turnover in Elderly Men and Women," *Medicine and Science in Sports and Exercise* 34, no. 1 (2002): 17–23.

Chapter 11

1 K. A. Grimm et al., "State-Specific Trends in Fruit and Vegetable Consumption among Adults—United States, 2000–2009," *Morbidity and Mortality Weekly Report* 59, no. 35 (2010): 1125–30.

2 "Are We Fooling Ourselves?" *Consumer Reports*, accessed March 10, 2012, www.consumerreports.org/health/healthy-living/diet-nutrition/diets-dieting/healthy-diet/overview/index.htm.

3 US Department of Agriculture and U.S. Department of Health and Human Services, *Dietary Guidelines for Americans, 2010*, 7th ed. (Washington, DC: US Government Printing Office, 2010).

4 US Department of Agriculture, "First Lady, Agriculture Secretary Launch *MyPlate* Icon as a New Reminder to Help Consumers Make Healthier Food Choices," news release, June 2, 2011, www.cnpp.usda.gov/Publications/MyPlate/PressRelease.pdf.

5 National Heart, Lung, and Blood Institute, "Portion Distortion and Serving Size," accessed March 10, 2012, www.nhlbi.nih.gov/health/public/heart/obesity/wecan/eat-right/distortion.htm.

6 Thomas L. Halton and Frank B. Hu, "The Effects of High Protein Diets on Thermogenesis, Satiety and Weight Loss: A Critical Review," *Journal of the American College of Nutrition*, 23, no. 5 (2004): 373–85.

7 Klaas R. Westerterp, "Diet Induced Thermogenesis," *Nutrition and Metabolism* 1 (2004): 5.

8 Christopher D. Gardner et al., "Comparison of the Atkins, Zone, Ornish, and LEARN Diets for Change in Weight and Related Risk Factors among Overweight Premenopausal Women: The A to Z Weight Loss Study: A Randomized Trial," *JAMA: The Journal of the American Medical Association* 297, no. 9 (2007): 969–77.

9 M. Garland et al., "The Relation Between Dietary Intake and Adipose Tissue Composition of Selected Fatty Acids in US Women," *American Journal of Clinical Nutrition* 67, no. 1 (1998): 25–30.

10 Organic Consumers Association, "Take Action! Tell USDA to Stop Factory Farm Organics," www.organicconsumers.org/nosb2.htm.

11 Environmental Working Group, "EWG's 2012 Shopper's Guide to Pesticides in Produce," accessed March 10, 2013, www.ewg.org/foodnews/summary.

12 Nicola M. McKeown et al., "Whole- and Refined-Grain Intakes Are Differentially Associated with Abdominal Visceral and Subcutaneous Adiposity in Healthy Adults: The Framingham Heart Study," *American Journal of Clinical Nutrition* 92, no. 5 (2010): 1165–71.

13 University of Sydney, Glycemic Index Home Page, accessed March 10, 2012, www.glycemicindex.com.

14 David S. Ludwig, "Artificially Sweetened Beverages: Cause for Concern," *Journal of the American Medical Association* 302, no. 22 (2009): 2477–78.

15 "Are We Fooling Ourselves?" *Consumer Reports,* accessed March 10, 2012, www.consumerreports.org/health/healthy-living/diet-nutrition/diets-dieting/healthy-diet/overview/index.htm.

16 Elizabeth A. Dennis et al., "Water Consumption Increases Weight Loss during a Hypocaloric Diet Intervention in Middle-Aged and Older Adults," *Obesity* 18, no. 2 (2010): 300–307.

17 Linda A. J. van Mierlo et al., "Suboptimal Potassium Intake and Potential Impact on Population Blood Pressure," *Archives of Internal Medicine* 170, no. 16 (2010): 1501–1502.

18 Rhonda S. Sebastian, Cecilia Wilkinson Enns, and Joseph D. Goldman, *Snacking Patterns of US Adults: What We Eat in America, NHANES 2007–2008*, Food Surveys Research Group Dietary Data Brief, no. 4 (Washington, DC: US Department of Agriculture, June 2011), http://ars.usda.gov/Services/docs.htm?docid=19476.

Index

Underscored page references indicate boxed text and tables.
Boldface references indicate illustrations and photographs.

A

Abdominal fat and obesity
  causes of, 162–63, 165, 166, 167, 245
  definition of, 141
  health problems from, 26, 27, 37, 41,
    140–41
  with metabolic syndrome, 35, 35, 100,
    101, 171
  reducing, with
    DHEA, 167
    mini-fast with exercise, 63, 209
    testosterone replacement, 166
Acorn squash
  Stuffed Squash with Turkey, 308
Aerobic exercise
  examples of, 89–90 (see also Walking)
  in fasting state, fat burning from, 118,
    196–98, 223, 256
  intensity level of, 90, 196, 197
  recommended duration and frequency
    of, 115, 118, 196–98
Alcohol consumption, 97, 249
Alli, 9
Almond butter and celery snack, 254
Almonds
  Chocolate-Almond Biscotti,
    334–35
  Rustic Peach and Almond Crisp,
    339
American diet, 95, 227–29
Amla, in Metabolic Essentials, 103
Anderson, Sue, 63
Animals, eating habits of, 3
Antidepressants, 175
Antipsychotic medications, 175
Appearance changes, for monitoring
  progress, 147–48
Appetite. See also Hunger
  vs. hunger, 52–53
  reducing, with
    breakfast skipping, 73
    general measures, 53, 118–20
    Mini-Fast Diet, 13–14

nutritional supplements, 13, 53, 120,
  121, 168–69
  specific foods, 53, 95, 232
  as survival tool, 117–18
Apples, for preventing overeating, 232
Arm circles, 215, 215
Armour natural thyroid, 159, 160
Arm-strengthening exercises, 214, 214–17,
  214–17
Arthritis, 24, 42–43
Artificial sweeteners, 246
Asparagus
  Asparagus Frittata, 261
Atkins diet, 7, 8, 14, 53, 236–37
Avocados
  Roasted Corn, Avocado, and Black
    Bean Salad, 269

B

Bacon. See Turkey bacon
Barbic, Bill, 188–89, 188
Bariatric surgery, 25
Basal body temperature
  how to test, 160
  thyroid function and, 159, 160
Basal metabolic rate (BMR), 76, 77, 139,
  157
  formula for determining, 78
  muscle increasing, 89, 208
Baxter, Gary, 201, 202
Beans
  for blood sugar control, 119
  Chicken Tacos with Corn and Black
    Bean Salsa, 304
  Cuban-Style Quinoa and Beans, 328
  Moroccan Lamb Chops with Garbanzo
    Relish, 298
  Roasted Corn, Avocado, and Black
    Bean Salad, 269
  Savory Bean Patties with Tahini Sauce,
    330–31
Bedtime, early, eating schedule and, 109

C

Cabbage
  Asian Grilled Tofu Steaks over Napa
    Slaw, 332–33
Caffeine. *See also* Coffee; Tea
  appetite-suppressing effect of, 118
  dehydration myth about, 249
  effects on exercise, 82, 91, 204
Calf raises, 222, 222
Caloric intake
  of Americans, overview of, 5, 5
  from beverages, 247
  from breakfast, 72–73
  breakfast skipping reducing, 56, 73,
    80, 226
  from snacks, 251, 256
Calorie burning
  from digestion, 77, 236
  from exercise, 15
  from muscle, 89
  for weight loss, 2
Calorie needs, equation for determining,
  78
Calorie restriction
  increasing longevity, 40
  from mini-fast, 12–13, 56, 73, 80,
    118, 226
  study on, 61–64
  for weight loss, 2, 7, 12, 46–47, 52
Calorie-rich foods, genetic attraction to,
  3, 4
Cancer
  DHEA and, 169
  from excess weight, 24, 37
  premature death from, 79
  prostate, 166, 169
  from sleep apnea, 41
Carbohydrates
  calorie burning from, 236
  consumption of, in American diet,
    5, 5
  diets restricting, 7, 8, 51, 53
  as energy source, 47–48, 50, 195, 240
  excess, converted to fat, 59
  exercise burning, 15, 58, 66–67
  glycemic index of, 53, 73, 76, 97, 119,
    241–43
  in Mini-Fast Diet eating plan, 242–43
  refined or simple, 241
    effect on blood sugar, 119, 242
    limiting, 97

Cardiovascular disease
  bariatric surgery reversing, 25
  hip size and, 140
  from obesity, 24, 28, 32–34, 140,
    245
  premature death from, 79
  risk factors for, 165, 171
  weight loss preventing, 34
Carney, Michael, 191, 257
Carnitine. *See* L-carnitine, in Ketosis
    Essentials
Carrots
  Oven-Roasted Chicken Breasts with
    Balsamic-Glazed Carrots, 299
Catfish
  Oven-Fried Catfish with Cajun Tartar
    Sauce, 320–21
Cauliflower
  Curried Chicken with Cauliflower and
    Zucchini, 302–3
Celery with nut butter, as snack, 254
Cereals, breakfast, 74, 75, 76
Cheerios, nutritional content of, 74, 75,
  76
Cheese
  Cheese Grits with Bacon, 264
  Cheesy Crab Casserole, 313
  Cheesy Onion Soup, 283
  Goat Cheese Soufflés, 262–63
  Grilled Two-Cheese on Whole Grain
    Bread, 282
  Raspberry Cheesecakes, 338
  reduced-fat, as snack, 254–55
  Spinach-Stuffed Eggplant Rollatini,
    326–27
Chicken
  Chicken and Grape Salad on Spring
    Greens, 275
  Chicken Provençal, 300
  Chicken Quesadillas, 279
  Chicken Tacos with Corn and Black
    Bean Salsa, 304
  Curried Chicken with Cauliflower and
    Zucchini, 302–3
  Oven-Roasted Chicken Breasts with
    Balsamic-Glazed Carrots,
    299
  Slow-Cooker Coq au Vin, 301
  Spice-Rubbed Chicken Thighs, 305
Chocolate
  Brownies, 341
  Chocolate-Almond Biscotti, 334–35

Holiday Cranberry-Turkey Meat Loaf,
306–7
Moussaka, 296–97
Open-Faced Mexican Stuffed-Turkey
Sandwiches, 276–77
Stuffed Squash with Turkey, 308
Turkey bacon
Cheese Grits with Bacon, 264
Turkey Bacon and Egg Sandwich,
260
Twisting crunches, 211, 211

U

Upper-body exercises, 208–9, 214,
214–17, 214–17

V

Valerian, as sleep aid, 178
Vegan diet, 85, 95, 240
Vegetable juice, 248
Vegetables. *See also specific vegetables*
in average American diet, 227
Beef and Vegetable Soup, 286
in eating plan, 96
fiber-rich, for blood sugar control, 119
potassium-rich, 250
for preventing overeating, 231–32
as snack, 254, 255
in Mini-Fast Diet eating plan, 242
Visceral fat
health risks from, 140–41
metabolic activity of, 26, 141
Vitamin D, in Metabolic Essentials, 103,
121

W

Waist-to-hip ratio, 139–42, 142, 143
Walking
as aerobic exercise, 89, 115
benefits of, 198–202, 209
intensity level of, 90
jogging with, 205–7, 207
pedometer for tracking, 200, 202–3
shoes for, 16
Wall pushups, 216, 216
Water drinking
before and after exercise, 91
during mini-fast, 82, 94
for weight loss, 248

Weigh-ins, regular, 137–38, 149, 155
Weight, social networks influencing,
124–25
Weight-bearing exercise, 89, 100
Weight gain. *See also* Obesity; Overweight
contributors to
artificial sweeteners, 246
bad habits, 136–37
diabetes treatments, 26
excessive screen time, 194
hormone replacement therapy, 164
polycystic ovary syndrome, 172
poor sleep, 176–79
prescription drugs, 26, 174–76
proton pump inhibitors, 42
sex hormones, 161–63
stress and emotional eating,
169–70
stress hormones, 166–67
testosterone deficiency in men, 165
thyroid disorders, 157–59, 161
underlying medical problems,
156–57, 179
diabetes risk from, 27
linked to metabolic syndrome and
cardiovascular disease, 28
Weight loss
from breakfast skipping, 118
calorie restriction for, 2, 7, 12, 46–47,
52
deciding to pursue, 132–33
diets for (*see* Diets)
drugs for, 9
failure of, 114
health benefits of
cancer prevention, 37
cardiovascular disease prevention,
32–34
diabetes control, 27–29
heartburn cure, 41–42
osteoarthritis prevention, 42–43
reversal of metabolic syndrome,
34–36, 102, 172, 173
reversal of nonalcoholic fatty liver
disease, 37–38
reversal of sleep apnea, 38, 40–41
instant willpower contract for, 131–32
maintaining (*see* Weight maintenance)
in men vs. women, 142
from mini-fast with exercise, 17, 63, 64,
65, 65–66, 102, 105, 112, 172,
173, 173, 209, 256

About the Author

Julian Whitaker, MD, is a graduate of Dartmouth College and Emory University Medical School. After postgraduate training in surgery at Emory, Dr. Whitaker worked with nutritional medicine pioneer Nathan Pritikin and in 1979 opened the Whitaker Wellness Institute. To date, more than 50,000 patients have been treated at the clinic, located in Newport Beach, California, with diet, exercise, targeted nutritional supplements, and safe, noninvasive therapies.

Dr. Whitaker is the author of 13 books, including *Reversing Heart Disease, Reversing Diabetes, Reversing Hypertension, The Pain Relief Breakthrough, The Memory Solution, Shed 10 Years in 10 Weeks,* and *Dr. Whitaker's Guide to Natural Healing.*

He is editor of the monthly newsletter *Health & Healing,* which has reached more than 4 million households since 1991. Dr. Whitaker is also a committed spokesman for freedom of choice in the medical arena and founder of the Freedom of Health Foundation.

Whitaker Wellness Institute
4321 Birch Street
Newport Beach, CA 92660
800-488-1500
whitakerwellness.com

About the Whitaker Wellness Institute

Founded by Julian Whitaker, MD, the Whitaker Wellness Institute in Newport Beach, California, is one of the oldest and most comprehensive alternative medicine clinics in the United States. Since 1979, more than 40,000 patients with heart disease, diabetes, obesity, and other serious diseases have come to the clinic seeking to get off prescription drugs, avoid surgery, and receive treatment with safe, proven therapies that are ignored by conventional physicians.

Patients participate in the clinic's 1-, 2-, or 3-week Back to Health Program, which involves extensive medical evaluation, diagnostic testing, and treatment. They receive a personalized nutritional supplement prescription, an individualized exercise program, and a therapeutic diet; and they undergo treatment with the unique therapies offered at Whitaker Wellness. These include enhanced external counterpulsation (EECP) to increase circulation and relieve angina; hyperbaric oxygen therapy to heal oxygen-starved tissues and reverse damage from stroke; laser and infrared light therapy to relieve pain and promote healing; and intravenous therapies for the treatment of a variety of conditions, including infections, vision problems, chronic fatigue, and Parkinson's disease.

During their stay at the clinic, patients also attend lectures by our physicians and informative, hands-on nutrition and cooking workshops. They participate in exercise and stress management classes and eat delicious, healthful meals prepared by our gourmet chef. They also enjoy the support and guidance of our caring, professional staff, as well as the encouragement and camaraderie of their fellow patients in their quest for optimal health.